Hatha Yoga Book 3

SHATKARMA

BIHAR SCHOOL OF YOGA

50 years

1963–2013

GOLDEN JUBILEE

WORLD YOGA CONVENTION 2013

GANGA DARSHAN, MUNGER, BIHAR, INDIA

23rd–27th October 2013

CONVERSATIONS ON THE SCIENCE OF YOGA

Hatha Yoga Book 3

SHATKARMA

From the teachings of
two great luminaries of the 20th century

Sri Swami Sivananda Saraswati
Sri Swami Satyananda Saraswati

Including answers from the satsangs of
Swami Niranjanananda Saraswati

Yoga Publications Trust, Munger, Bihar, India

Published by Yoga Publications Trust
First edition 2013

ISBN: 978-93-81620-61-8

Publisher and distributor: Yoga Publications Trust, Ganga Darshan, Munger, Bihar, India.

Website: www.biharyoga.net
www.rikhiapeeth.net

Printed at Aegean Offset Printers, Greater Noida

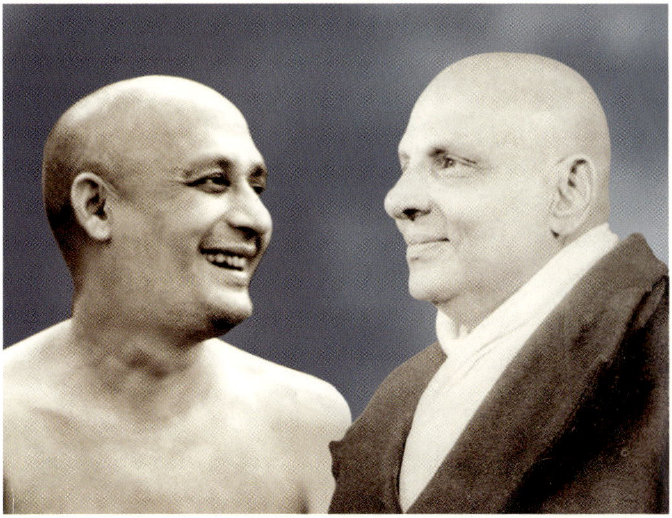

Dedication

In humility we offer this dedication to
Swami Sivananda Saraswati, who initiated
Swami Satyananda Saraswati into the secrets of yoga
and to our guru Sri Swami Satyananda Saraswati
who continues to inspire and guide us
on our spiritual journey.

Swami Niranjan

Contents

Preface

CONVERSATIONS ON THE SCIENCE OF YOGA

Conversations on the Science of Yoga is an encyclopaedic series which brings together the collected teachings of two generations of masters – Swami Sivananda Saraswati of Rishikesh and Swami Satyananda Saraswati of Munger. Satsangs given by Swami Niranjanananda Saraswati on his numerous national and international tours also provide the answers to many questions on this vast subject. These luminaries represent a living tradition in which the eternal knowledge and wisdom of yoga has been passed from guru to disciple in a dynamic continuum from the early twentieth century to the first decades of the twenty-first century.

The series consists of sets of books which present the timeless culture of yoga topic by topic, in question and answer format. In this way, complex and profound subjects such as karma yoga, hatha yoga and bhakti yoga, are presented in clear, simple language. These conversations on yoga reflect an ancient and enduring approach to the transmission of wisdom, in which spiritual aspirants seek answers to their questions at the feet of the guru.

Many of the answers also include verses from the various relevant scriptures, connecting the modern experience with the classical tradition. It is through the lives and teachings of the masters that the scriptures are correctly and intuitively interpreted for each generation, ensuring that the light of these revelations continues to illumine and inspire the hearts and minds of all who aspire for spiritual upliftment.

Conversations on the Science of Yoga has been compiled from the rich archive of satsangs and writings, both published and unpublished, which is held at the Bihar School of Yoga, Munger. The organization of this material into the major branches of yoga and related topics creates a unique interpretation of the classical yogic sciences for the benefit of humanity in the modern era. Deeply founded in tradition, the teachings are both systematic and practical, addressing the needs of individuals and society at a time when adjustment to constant change is placing unprecedented pressure on people all over the world.

The Bihar Yoga tradition

Bihar School of Yoga is ideally placed to produce this major contribution to yogic literature. Founded in 1963 by Swami Satyananda Saraswati, the system known in India as Bihar Yoga and internationally as Satyananda Yoga, seamlessly integrates all facets of the yogic tradition, including the various branches of yoga, the philosophies which are fundamental to the yogic culture and the dynamism of self-

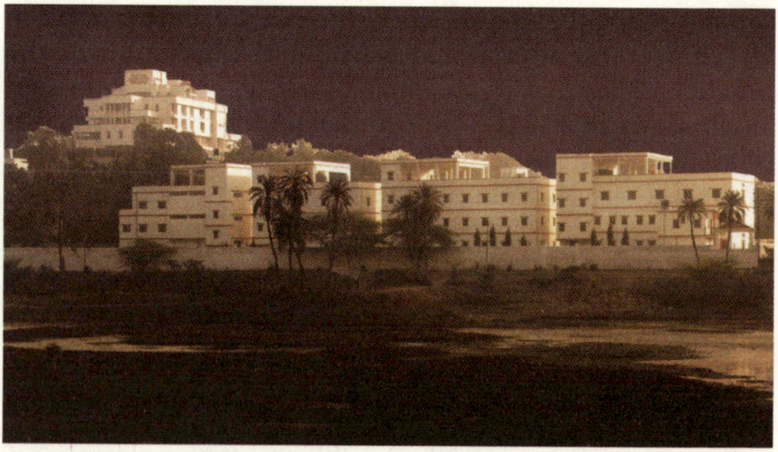

realized preceptors which ensures that the teachings remain fresh and relevant in any age. This all-inclusive approach means that yogic practices are available as tools for holistic life management, while other *vidyas*, spiritual sciences, such as Tantra, Vedanta and Samkhya provide a broad philosophical base. Emerging from this living tradition, *Conversations on the Science of Yoga* is a unique and precious offering to humanity.

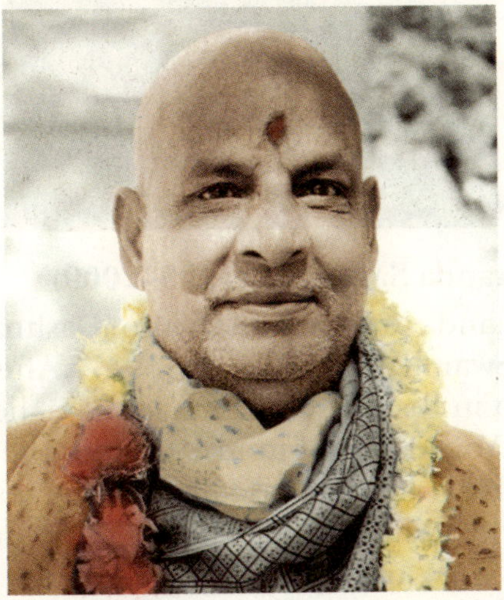

Swami Sivananda Saraswati (1887–1963)

Swami Sivananda was a towering spiritual force in the yogic renaissance which developed in India in the first half of the twentieth century. After serving as a doctor in Malaya, he returned to India to pursue his spiritual aspirations, and in 1924 was initiated into Dashnami sannyasa in Rishikesh. He founded the Divine Life Society, toured India extensively, wrote hundreds of books and inspired thousands around the world to practise yoga and lead a divine life. Swami Sivananda's eightfold path of yoga – serve, love, give, purify, do good, be good, meditate, realize – expresses his philosophy of service to humanity and continues to guide the work of the Bihar School of Yoga.

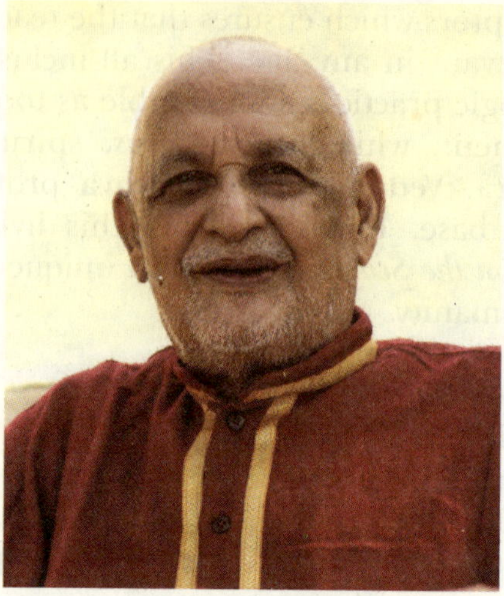

Swami Satyananda Saraswati (1923–2009)

Swami Satyananda was initiated into Dashnami sannyasa by his guru Swami Sivananda, in 1947. After serving his guru's mission in Rishikesh for twelve years, he founded the International Yoga Fellowship in 1956 and the Bihar School of Yoga in 1963. From that base he took the teachings to the rest of the world, fulfilling the mandate of his guru to 'spread yoga from door to door and shore to shore.'

Through his genius and compassion, many ancient, complex and esoteric practices were systematized, simplified and made available to people of all ages, cultures and creeds. Swami Satyananda's blend of charisma and pragmatism attracted multitudes of devotees wherever he went, giving rise to a global movement and creating a far-reaching network of ashrams, yoga centres and teachers. Meanwhile, the headquarters in Bihar continued to expand its many programs, including the publishing division, producing numerous books that both preserve and disseminate the incredibly rich seam of practical wisdom which flows through this lineage.

In 1988 Swami Satyananda renounced his mission in order to live as a paramahamsa sannyasin, performing higher spiritual and vedic sadhanas in an isolated location. During this chapter of his life, he also realized his guru's teaching of 'serve, love, give', by establishing Sivananda Math, an organization dedicated to raising the living standards of the weaker and underprivileged sectors of society.

At midnight on 5 December 2009, Sri Swami Satyananda Saraswati attained mahasamadhi.

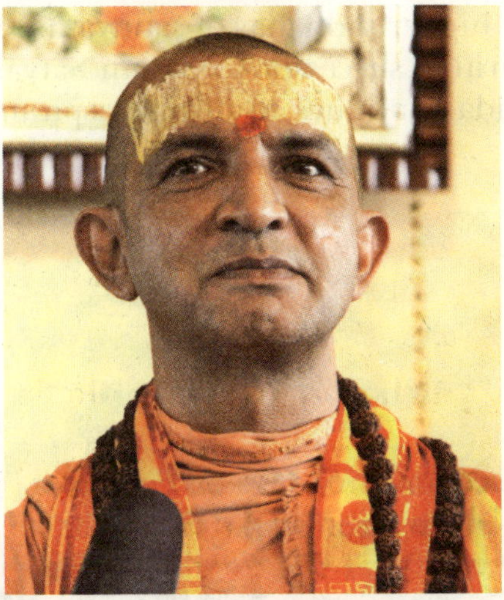

Swami Niranjanananda Saraswati (1960)

A yogi from earliest childhood, Swami Niranjanananda joined the Bihar School of Yoga in 1964 and was initiated into Dashnami sannyasa in 1971. At the age of eleven he was sent to live abroad by his guru Swami Satyananda, giving him direct experience and understanding of people from a vast array of cultures and walks of life. These years instilled in him a rare, cross-cultural insight into human nature, enabling him to communicate and interact with the international community with familiarity, ease and humour.

Combined with his depth of spiritual and yogic knowledge, this background equipped Swami Niranjanananda to guide the Bihar School of Yoga and the international yoga movement from 1983 until 2008, when he began handing over the administration to the next generation. During this time he also authored many classic books on yoga, tantra and the upanishads and founded Bihar Yoga Bharati, the world's first yoga university, while continuing extensive national and international touring.

Following retirement from his role at the Bihar School of Yoga, Swami Niranjanananda established Sannyasa Peeth for the development and training of sannyasins, and for his own pursuit of the higher sadhanas of sannyasa.

As the spiritual successor to Swami Satyananda, Swami Niranjanananda continues to inspire aspirants around the world.

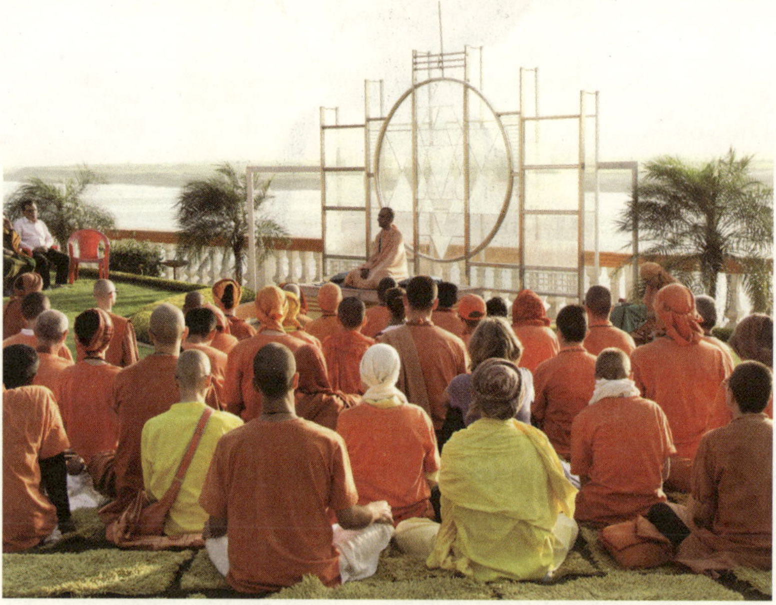

Yoga is not a philosophy, it is a practical science. Philosophy gives you knowledge, yoga gives you experience. This is the beauty of yoga. That experience is a manifestation of your inner being.

—*Swami Satyananda Saraswati*

Introduction

> To transcend the body does not mean to just forget about it. One has to purify it. Therefore, these six kriyas of hatha yoga are necessary for spiritual aspirants.
>
> —*Swami Satyananda*

The yogic techniques for cleansing the inner body, known as the *shatkarmas*, are the original practices of hatha yoga. The word simply means 'six actions', hence they are sometimes referred to as the *shatkriyas*, which has the same meaning. The purpose of the shatkarmas within the hatha yoga tradition is to purify the body in preparation for higher sadhanas, particularly pranayama. Their effect on both general health and specific ailments is therapeutic and also preventative. Unfortunately, this unique system is little known, even amongst practitioners of hatha yoga, who tend to focus on asanas. In *Hatha Yoga Book 3: Shatkarma*, three modern yogic masters present a rare wealth of knowledge on the subject, leaving no doubt as to the potential benefits that would flow from widespread appreciation and practise of these kriyas.

At first glance the shatkarmas may seem to have nothing to do with spiritual goals. The yogis of ancient times, however, understood the importance of physical health when in pursuit of spiritual heights, recognizing disease as an obstacle to spiritual evolution. A weak body cannot practise advanced asanas, whose purpose is to stimulate, activate and direct the energy of specific pranas and chakras. A weak body cannot sustain the lengthy practise of pranayamas with high ratios of inhalation, retention and exhalation of the breath. A weak body cannot sit comfortably and upright in meditative poses for hours with one-pointed focus on the object of meditation.

The shatkarma techniques, therefore, were developed as the starting point for the attainment of a strong, resilient constitution: possessing excellent health, a yogi could practise extensive sadhanas without interruption or distraction due to bodily disorders. This pragmatic, commonsense approach to spiritual life is characteristic of hatha yoga, which gives step by step guidelines for the progress of all sincere aspirants. In the words of Swami Sivananda, "Before awakening the kundalini, one must have purity of body, purification of nadis, purity of mind and purity of intellect. For the purification of the body, the hatha yoga shatkarmas are prescribed."

The body-mind connection

The regions acted on most directly by many of the shatkarmas are the respiratory and digestive systems. These two systems are responsible for much of the body's energy intake and waste removal. If they are compromised due to congestion or imbalance, the functioning of the entire body-mind is compromised. A respiratory system clogged with mucus cannot breathe properly, adversely affecting respiration, pranic strength and the brain. A digestive system suffering from irritable bowel syndrome, hyperacidity, constipation, piles or other disorders cannot efficiently deliver the nutrients and prana needed for maintaining the physical and mental structure. Such conditions also cause pain and discomfort.

The effect of any disorders in these systems has major implications for the mind as well as the body, as the relationship of the body with the mind is two-way. This entwined relationship of the body-mind is a key concept underpinning hatha yoga, the aim of which is to enable and facilitate mind management by optimizing and balancing the energy flows in the body. Poor health causes blockages to the flow of prana, hence the focus of hatha yoga on physical health, starting with the practice of shatkarmas. According to Swami Niranjanananda, "Cleansing the body directly affects how the mind is experienced. If one's internal body is unclean, a certain disharmony is felt in the mind. Recognizing this particular tendency, hatha yoga developed the shatkarma practices."

Significantly, the final two shatkarma practices are intended to cleanse the brain, for the brain is also a type of container which is continually filled with material that needs 'digesting'. Just as the digestive and respiratory systems generate waste which leaves a residue, so too the brain, as it becomes clogged from too much thinking, intrusive memories, and in modern times, sensory over-stimulation. How can the brain be cleansed? Hatha yoga has a way. For this subtle purpose, the shatkarmas include the practices of *kapalbhati*, the frontal brain cleansing breath, and *trataka*, a technique of steady gazing. With these two unique practices, the role of the shatkarmas is complete, and the yogi possesses not only a pure body, but also a clear, concentrated mind.

Health care revolution

Modern health systems are high tech and high expense, and while medical advances have revolutionized health care and relieved much suffering from acute and chronic diseases, there has been a concurrent increase in lifestyle-related illnesses, such as asthma, diabetes, heart disease, cancer and obesity. Even in affluent countries, health care structures are overloaded and cannot meet the needs of the people. A mentality of dependence is part of the problem, as health management has become an incredibly complex area of expertise instead of being part of the fundamental knowledge of an individual, a family or small community.

By contrast, the hatha yoga shatkarmas offer a do-it-yourself health management system for healing, maintaining and enhancing the functioning of the body's systems, including the brain. Swami Satyananda explains the role of the shatkarmas in caring for oneself with a simple analogy: "As with a car, one's body requires constant attention and care. It requires regular servicing and cleaning of its major organs and parts. The hatha yoga shatkarmas are prescribed for the constant care and cleaning of the body and mind."

In the current era, yoga has come out of seclusion and into the mainstream. The use of asanas for flexibility and toning the body is well recognized. The use of yogic relaxation, breathing techniques and meditation for stress management is accepted and on the increase. The shatkarmas also have a major role to play in improving the quality of life and giving people a way of becoming more independent in personal health care. For various reasons, however, they have not yet been popularized, in spite of their pivotal role in traditional hatha yoga.

Why has the use of shatkarmas been so limited to date? Whilst other aspects of yoga have become global, the shatkarmas have not been widely disseminated by the gurus and teachers who have spread hatha yoga. Satyananda Yoga is a notable exception. Due to innovations by Swami Satyananda, the contribution of this tradition to adapting and developing the shatkarmas for general use is unsurpassed.

The shatkarmas in Satyananda Yoga

The shatkarma practices range from those that are easy to do on a daily basis to others which are complex and for occasional practice under supervision. The classical hatha yoga texts give minimal descriptions of how to perform the shatkarmas, emphasizing that they should be practised under the guidance of a qualified guru. They were written for dedicated hatha yogis, a highly specialized group with advanced technical knowledge of the subject, which was kept secret from the general public. Just as an astronaut would not trust the average person to fly their spaceship, the highly accomplished hatha yogis protected the novice from the power of the practices by only revealing the details to qualified disciples. Given the mission of spreading yoga from 'door to door and shore to shore', Swami Satyananda analyzed the vast array of yogic techniques, including the shatkarmas, with the intention of transforming yoga into a widely available system able to benefit the maximum number of people. As a result, just as virtually anyone can learn to ride a bicycle or drive a car, a selection of the shatkarmas has been made accessible to all who are prepared to undertake some basic training.

Notable among these are the practices of *jala neti*, cleansing the nostrils with water, and *shankhaprakshalana*, the complete intestinal wash. The methods devised by Swami Satyananda mean that these two key practices can easily be taught to yoga students by their teacher, and safely practised at home. The shatkarma techniques of kapalbhati, agnisar kriya (traditionally known as vahnisara dhauti) and trataka are routinely included in the integral yoga classes taught by Satyananda Yoga teachers around the world. This selection is all that is needed for general purposes.

Within the Satyananda Yoga tradition, still other shatkarma practices are reserved for supervised therapeutic use: for example, *vastra dhauti*, cleansing the upper digestive tract with cloth, for asthma, and *moola shodhana*, anal cleansing, for severe constipation. From the remainder of the traditional shatkarmas, several are not suitable or appropriate for the modern lifestyle: some must be performed while standing in fast flowing, pure water, which has sadly become an environmental rarity; others require lengthy training to develop the necessary muscular control, and the effects can be achieved more simply by the practices Swami Satyananda has focused on.

Hatha Yoga Book 3: Shatkarma is not intended as a practice manual, rather it is a unique compilation of questions and answers derived from the discourses and writings of Swami Sivananda, Swami Satyananda and Swami Niranjanananda, including pertinent quotes from the hatha yoga scriptures. As such it is a much-needed and unique contribution to the literature available on the shatkarmas, drawing on the direct experience and profound insight of these enlightened yogic masters of the twentieth and twenty-first centuries. There is a chapter on each of the shatkarma categories, presenting a comprehensive picture of the techniques, their purposes, benefits and contra-indications. Additionally, the effects of the shatkarmas on the *pranamaya kosha*, or energy body, and guidelines for shatkarma sadhana are included. With the publication of this volume, the fundamental importance of the shatkarmas within hatha yoga, and their potential as a group of practices becomes clear to the modern practitioner.

Note

Hatha Yoga Book 3: Shatkarma is not an instruction book. Shatkarmas should always be learned from a qualified teacher with understanding of contra-indications and precautions.

Detailed technical instructions for the practicable shatkarmas are included in Swami Satyananda's practice guide, *Asana Pranayama Mudra Bandha*, as well as in various specialized books published by Yoga Publications Trust.

1

Understanding the Shatkarmas

DEFINITION AND CLASSIFICATION

What are the hatha yoga shatkarmas?

Swami Satyananda: Hatha yoga, as described in the early Yoga Upanishads, was made up of the shatkarmas and is a precise and systematic science. *Shat* means 'six' and *karma* means 'action'; the shatkarmas consist of six groups of purification practices. The aim of hatha yoga, and therefore of the shatkarmas, is to create harmony between the two major pranic flows, ida and pingala, resulting in physical and mental purification and balance. There are six main groups of *shatkarmas*, or yogic cleansers:

1. *Neti*: nasal cleansing
2. *Dhauti*: cleansing of the digestive tract
3. *Nauli*: rolling the abdominal muscles
4. *Basti*: colon cleaning
5. *Kapalbhati*: purification and vitalization of the frontal brain
6. *Trataka*: blinkless gazing at one point.

How are the hatha yoga cleansing techniques classified?

Swami Satyananda: There are only six categories of these practices, but within each there are a variety of practices.

Neti has four practices: *jala neti*, passing warm saline water through the nose, *sutra neti*, passing a soft thread through the nose, *ghrita neti*, passing ghee, clarified butter through the nose, and *dugdha neti*, passing milk through the nose.

Dhauti is divided into four parts. According to the *Gheranda Samhita* they are called *antar*, internal, dhauti, *danta*, teeth, dhauti, *hrid*, cardiac, dhauti and *moola shodhana*, rectal cleaning.

Antar dhauti is further divided into four practices: *vatsara dhauti*, expelling air through the anus, *varisara dhauti*, evacuating a large quantity of water through the bowels, *vahnisara dhauti*, rapid expansion and contraction of the abdomen (agnisar kriya), *bahishkrita dhauti*, washing the rectum.

Hrid dhauti is divided into three practices: *danda dhauti*, inserting a soft banana stem into the stomach, *vastra dhauti*, swallowing a long thin strip of cloth, *vaman dhauti*, regurgitating the contents of the stomach.

The last practice of dhauti, moola shodhana can be performed in two ways. It is done either by inserting a turmeric root or the middle finger into the anus.

Nauli is a practice in which the abdominal muscles are isolated and churned. It has three practices. When the muscles are isolated to the right, it is *dakshina* nauli, to the left, *vama* nauli and in the middle it is *madhyama* nauli.

Basti is divided into two parts: *jala*, water, basti and *sthala*, dry, basti. In *jala basti* water is sucked into the large intestine through the anus and then expelled. In *sthala basti* air is sucked into the large intestine.

Kapalbhati has three practices: *vatakrama kapalbhati*, which is similar to bhastrika pranayama, *vyutkrama kapalbhati*, sucking water in through the nose and expelling it through the mouth, and *sheetkrama kapalbhati*, sucking water in through the mouth and expelling it through the nose.

Trataka is steady and continuous gazing at a point of concentration. It has two practices: *antar*, internal, and *bahir*, external, trataka.

These six fundamental cleansing techniques are a most important aspect of hatha yoga and are the original practices of hatha yoga. Today, however, asana and pranayama are more widely known and few people are proficient in the shatkarmas.

How are the shatkarmas classified according to the *Gheranda Samhita*?

Swami Niranjanananda: Shatkarmas are those practices which regulate the functioning of the internal organs and make them free from disease. Sage Gheranda lists them as:

1. *Dhauti kriya*: The first practice is *dhauti*, cleansing of the stomach and alimentary canal or digestive tract. There are four types of dhauti: antar dhauti, danta dhauti, hrid dhauti and moola shodhana. Three methods are used: with water, with cloth or with air. These techniques help to remove many stomach ailments. Indigestion and other abdominal disorders such as constipation, irritable bowel syndrome and hyperacidity can be cured by practising dhauti.

2. *Basti kriya*: The second practice is *basti*, yogic enema. In basti, water is sucked up through the anus and kept in the large intestine for some time. The water does not enter the small intestine, but remains in the large intestine. After some time the water is expelled, just as in a regular enema. The only difference is that in an enema a tube is used. Basti is more natural and more appropriate. When an enema is given, excessive force may be applied, resulting in scratches inside the body with the potential for internal injury and bleeding. The waste matter is toxic, so when it comes into contact with a wound, infection can result. Therefore, yoga recommends basti instead of an enema. However, first the practice has to be perfected, and while learning the technique a rubber tube or catheter is required.

3. *Neti kriya*: The third practice is *neti*, nasal cleansing. It is a simple practice. Sage Gheranda describes the variation in which a thread is passed through the nostrils. Alternatively, water is poured in one nostril and flows out the other. The benefits are experienced as soon as the practice is done, as it clears the nasal passages and sinuses.

Shatkarma practices

DHAUTI	**Antar dhauti** (internal)	Vatsara (air) Varisara (shankha-prakshalana) Vahnisara (agnisara kriya) Bahishkrita (rectal cleaning)
	Danta dhauti (head)	Dantamoola (teeth) Jihva (tongue) Karnarandhra (ears) Kapalrandhra (frontal sinuses)
	Hrid dhauti (cardiac)	Danda (stick) Vaman (kunjal & vyaghra kriya) Vastra (cloth)
	Moola shodhana (anal)	
BASTI	**Jala** (water) **Sthala** (dry)	
NETI	**Jala** (water) **Sutra** (thread)	
LAULIKI (NAULI)	**Madhyama** (middle) **Vama** (left) **Dakshina** (right) **Bhramara** (abdomen)	
TRATAKA	**Bahiranga** (external) **Antaranga** (internal)	
KAPALBHATI	**Vatakrama** (breathing) **Vyutkrama** (reversed) **Sheetkrama** (cooling)	

Neti is beneficial for people suffering from sinusitis, rhinitis, headache, migraine or constant frontal headache, and minor ailments of the eyes, ears and throat.

4. *Lauliki kriya*: The fourth practice is lauliki, which is also called nauli. It is a powerful technique which massages and strengthens all the abdominal organs. It should be practised by those suffering from indigestion, loss of appetite or intestinal worms. It is also useful for removing excess *vata* or wind.

5. *Trataka*: The fifth practice is *trataka,* steady gazing, which is useful for removing eye defects and balancing the nervous system. It can, for example, help to remove nervous tics or uncontrolled nervous activity such as one eye blinking quickly. Trataka can relieve eyestrain, short sightedness, far sightedness, myopia and other eye defects in a healthy body. Experience has also shown that with the practice of trataka alone, many people no longer need to wear spectacles.

6. *Kapalbhati*: The sixth practice is *kapalbhati.* This is a breathing technique that clears the head and can help to remove defects of the lungs. The trachea or windpipe becomes free from disease and the blood is purified, as a greater volume of oxygen is taken in and a greater volume of carbon dioxide is expelled. Kapalbhati is useful for correcting imbalances of the autonomic nervous system and mental disorders. It is also useful for a weakened memory. Research conducted in an American university found that memory retention in older people can be improved by practising pawanmuktasana part one and kapalbhati for six months.

Do the hatha yoga scriptures differ in their descriptions of the cleansing techniques?

Swami Satyananda: According to *Gheranda Samhita* and *Hatha Yoga Pradipika* there are six groups of yogic cleansing techniques. They are called the shatkarmas and are as follows: dhauti, basti, neti, nauli, trataka and kapalbhati. In the *Gheranda Samhita* the sixth shatkarma is given as bhalbhati. Often kapalbhati and bhalbhati are regarded as the same practice with different names but actually they differ. *Hatharatnavali* describes eight purificatory processes, saying (1:25):

Atra vayam gurusampradaayaanusaarena naulyaadyashta-karmaani broomah.
Chakrirnaulirdhauti rneti rvasti rgajakarinee.
Trotanam mastakabhaatih karmaanyashtau prachakshate.

Now I will speak on the eight karmas according to the guru tradition: chakri, nauli, dhauti, neti, basti, gajakarani, trataka and mastakabhati (kapalbhati); these are said to be eight purificatory processes.

PURPOSE

Should everyone practise the shatkarmas?

Swami Sivananda: Everyone need not practise these techniques. Those who have too much phlegm in the body should practise these kriyas. Learn them under an expert hatha yogi. Hatha yoga is not the goal. It is only a means to an end. One should take to raja yoga after possessing good health.

What is the ultimate purpose of the shatkarmas?

Swami Satyananda: Hatha yoga says that shatkarmas must be practised first. The purpose of emphasizing shatkarmas is to prepare a base for the higher practices of pranayama. Shatkarmas purify the whole system and remove blockages on the paths of ida and pingala nadis. When there are no blockages on these paths, the breath in both the nostrils flows systematically. When the left nostril flows, it means ida is active. When the right nostril flows, it means pingala is active. When the left nostril flows, it means the mind is dominant. When the right nostril flows, it means the pranas are dominant. The flow of breath in the alternate nostrils indicates the activity of the parasympathetic and sympathetic nervous systems. The practices of shatkarma ultimately bring about a union of ida and pingala, and when ida and pingala unite, sushumna awakens.

What is the role of the shatkarmas in the overall scheme of yoga?

Swami Niranjanananda: In the proper application of yoga, everyone must go through the practices of hatha yoga, including the cleansing techniques, to rid the body of the toxicity accumulated at both the gross and subtle levels.

The yogic tradition says, and it is implied in the *Yoga Sutras* of Sage Patanjali, that before the commencement of raja yoga or ashtanga yoga practices, the practices of hatha yoga must be perfected. Without perfection in hatha yoga, one cannot enter into raja yoga. Life, and one's needs, must be looked at from two perspectives.

What is one's need? Why does one come to yoga? If someone comes to yoga for temporary gain, like eradication of a problem, illness, disease, stress or tension, and yoga is used as an alternative method of healing, it makes no difference what type of yoga is practised. Anything can be practised: the quality of health and life, body and mind can be improved, and after achieving one's aspirations, the practice of yoga can be forgotten about completely. That is one way of looking at yoga, and it is the trend which most people follow.

The other method is to decide whether yoga is going to become one's discipline in life or not. If it is taken on as a discipline, it becomes a way of transcending the limitations of one's senses, mind and personality. If one is aiming for this type of qualitative transformation to enhance the process of evolution, and for an inner awakening which brings one closer to the world in which one lives with other people, yoga must be practised with an appropriate sankalpa and applied properly in life – not merely taking one grain here, one grain there, and another grain there.

One must also begin the training, the self-education of the mind, as the state of physical purity and detoxification leads to a balance between the physical energies and the mental energies, *prana shakti* and *chitta shakti*, the vital force and the mental force, the solar force and the lunar force, the yang and the yin. They both merge in ajna chakra. The purpose of hatha yoga is to awaken these twin forces within and bring about balance in their functions.

Hatha yoga is a specific branch of yoga whose purpose is to cleanse the pathways of prana shakti: this cleaning is known as *nadi shuddhi*. The cleansing techniques of hatha yoga, numbering six, clean the entire system from the head right down to the perineum, including the oesophagus, the stomach, the small intestine and the large intestine: it is a complete cleaning system for the internal body. After the body has been cleansed with the practices of neti, dhauti and basti, pranayama is taught to ensure that the prana shakti goes through those *nadis*, those channels that have been purified. Concentration is taught, and activation of the chakras is stimulated through specific kriyas.

What comes after neti, dhauti and basti? Kapalbhati: kapalphati is not just one practice of pranayama, it is a series of methods to control the movement of prana in the body. Trataka: trataka is the simplest way to focus the mind without having to fight and struggle with oneself. And nauli: is the specific kriya to activate a particular psychic centre in the space of manipura chakra, the storehouse of prana shakti, the generating source of prana shakti.

Along with these cleansing techniques and specific kriyas, are the *bandhas,* energy locks, and *mudras,* techniques to divert the flow of energy in the body. They must be learnt, for only then can one derive the actual, appropriate benefits from the practices of raja yoga. The yogic tradition states clearly that before the practice of raja yoga, one must perfect hatha yoga. And before attempting to practise the higher yogas, perfect raja yoga – it is a sequence, there is a process.

People like to jump the gun, that's the problem. If you are willing to make yoga into a discipline of life, don't jump the gun, follow the system. If the system is followed, attainments and achievements in life will definitely be positive.

What is the role of the shatkarmas in the system of yoga outlined in *Gheranda Samhita*?

Swami Niranjanananda: In *Gheranda Samhita, saptanga yoga*, seven limbs of yoga, are described. These seven limbs or states are: *shodhana,* purity, *dridhata,* firmness, *sthairya,* steadiness, *dhairya,* patience, *laghava,* lightness of body, *pratyaksha,* acquiring subtle perception, and *nirlipta,* non-involvement. The purpose of the shatkarmas is directly related to the first two of these states.

Purity of the body, shodhana, is the goal of the first three shatkarmas. Sage Gheranda gives a detailed description of this process. The practices purify the gross and subtle bodies and bring them into a controlled, harmonious and healthy state.

The aim of the fourth, fifth and sixth shatkarmas is to provide energy which can be used to achieve dridhata, firmness. In this state, stimulation of the digestive fire occurs automatically.

What are some of the subtle effects of the cleansing practices?

Swami Niranjanananda: The first three practices, neti, dhauti and basti, purify the physical structure in preparation for the awakening of the subtle energies in the body. The fourth practice, nauli, stimulates the source of energy and balances the entire pranic body, *the pranamaya kosha*. The fifth practice, kapalbhati, is a way of cleansing the mind, the psychic body and the pranic body from impurities and the accumulation of samskaras and impressions that clutter the mind. The sixth practice, trataka, is a technique of dharana which focuses the mind on one point or one object of concentration.

How important are the shatkarmas in hatha yoga sadhana?

Swami Satyananda: Yogic science gives as much importance to certain cleansing processes as it does to asanas or pranayamas. They are important from the point of view of physical and mental health, and these simple techniques are also highly valuable in healing internal disorders.

Without regular cleansing of the body's internal systems, maximum benefits from yoga practices will not be gained. Without purification of the body one will not be ready for the higher practices of yoga. These practices are used before pranayama and other higher yoga practices in order to purify the body of toxins and to ensure safe and successful progression along the spiritual path. When the body is free, the mind also functions properly. In *Hatha Yoga Pradipika* (2:23) it states:

> *Karmashatkamidam gopyam ghatashodhanakaarakam.*
> *Vichitragunasandhaayi poojyate yogipungavaih.*
>
> These shatkarmas which effect purification of the body are secret. They have manifold, wondrous results and are held in high esteem by eminent yogis.

What is the best way to maintain a healthy bodily system?

Swami Satyananda: As with a car, one's body requires constant attention and care. It requires regular servicing and cleaning of its major organs and parts. The hatha yoga shatkarmas are prescribed for the constant care and cleaning of the body and mind.

By the practices of neti, dhauti, nauli, basti, kapalbhati and trataka, one is able to maintain the body against the wear and tear of life. Excess waste materials that build up in the different parts of the body are eliminated.

How can one increase one's capacity for sadhana and for life's activities?

Swami Satyananda: The shatkarmas specifically increase the vital capacity of the practitioner. They were never designed for therapy alone, but to create harmony in the body and mind and to prepare one for further practices. As they bring about smooth and perfect functioning of the bodily systems, it is inevitable that through their practice the mind will become free from turbulence and disturbances and thus be better able to concentrate and move towards dhyana.

These practices are necessary for those people who want to have good spiritual practice like concentration and sitting in an asana for two or three hours, as for these sadhanas, the body must be pure. If there is hyperacidity, and one sits for meditation, one is only going to have those experiences which are instigated by hyperacidity. The experiences will not be spiritual experiences. They will be hyperacidity experiences.

The effects of shatkarma can be summed up in one word – purification. When the systems of the body have been purified, the overall result is that energy can flow freely through the body. One's capacity to work, think, digest, taste, feel and experience increases, and greater awareness develops. It is no wonder that the yogis who have achieved perfection and know the real extent of human capacity, regard the shatkarmas with great esteem.

Why is physical purification needed for spiritual progress?

Swami Satyananda: There are people who say, "Oh, I am spiritual. I don't care about the physical body; hatha yoga only makes one body-minded." What is this nonsense? When someone is spiritually-minded and sits for meditation, awareness of the body comes with great force. One may even have to go to a doctor if the body can't be controlled without help. To transcend the body does not mean to just forget about it. One has to purify it. Therefore, these six kriyas of hatha yoga, neti, dhauti, basti, nauli, kapalbhati and trataka, are necessary for spiritual aspirants.

What effect do the shatkarmas have on the doshas?

Swami Satyananda: The shatkarmas are used to balance the three *doshas* or humours in the body: *kapha*, mucus; *pitta*, bile; and *vata*, wind. According to both ayurveda and hatha yoga, an imbalance in the doshas results in illness.

How do the shatkarmas balance the body?

Swami Niranjanananda: Through the shatkarmas, harmonization of ida and pingala, the two main flows of prana, is established, resulting in physical and mental purity and balance. The shatkarmas also balance vata, pitta, and kapha, the three disorders created in the body. According to ayurveda and hatha yoga, any imbalance in these three disorders gives rise to disease. Additionally, the shatkarmas are used before pranayama and other higher practices of yoga so that the body becomes free from disease and does not create any obstacles on the spiritual path. In *Gheranda Samhita* (1:10) it is written:

> *Shatkarmanaa shodhanam cha aasanena bhaveddridham;*
> *Mudrayaa sthirataa chaiva pratyaahaarena dheerataa.*
>
> Through shatkarmas purification of body and through asanas firmness, through mudras steadiness and through pratyahara patience is achieved.

Why does *Gheranda Samhita* place so much importance on the practice of shatkarmas as preparation for pranayama?

Swami Niranjanananda: In the yogic tradition, shatkarmas are embedded in the study of pranayama. This is not so clear when one begins to study the *Gheranda Samhita* as the first chapter is devoted to so many variations of shatkarmas. At that stage one has no perspective, so shatkarma tends to be practised as an end in itself. However, by the time the chapter on pranayama is reached, under the guidance of an experienced teacher a different perspective will have been acquired.

King Chandakapali asks Sage Gheranda, "How are the nadis purified? Please teach me all about this." His guru replies, "The vital air cannot enter the nadis while they are full of impurities, so how can pranayama be accomplished? How can there be knowledge of the tattwas? Therefore, one should first purify the nadis and only then practise pranayama. This purification of the nadis is of two kinds: samanu and nirmanu. *Samanu* is done as a mental process with mantras, *nirmanu* is done by physical cleansing. The shatkarmas (i.e. nirmanu) have already been taught, now listen . . ."

BENEFITS

Why are shatkarmas important for kundalini awakening?

Swami Sivananda: Shatkarmas are intended for the purification of the body. When the nadis are impure, kundalini cannot pass from mooladhara to sahasrara chakra. Purification of nadis is effected through pranayama. Before practising pranayama, the body must be purified by the shatkarmas.

Why is it important to cleanse the internal body?

Swami Niranjanananda: Cleaning the body internally is as important as cleaning the body externally. How would it feel not to clean one's mouth or brush the teeth for one week? If you do not know, try it. How would it feel not to go to the toilet for a week? If you do not know, try it.

Cleaning the body is necessary in order to experience harmony and balance inside. Cleansing the body directly affects how the mind is experienced. If one's internal body is unclean, a certain disharmony is felt in the mind. Recognizing this particular tendency, hatha yoga developed these shatkarma practices, but for a certain purpose.

How does the accumulation of bodily waste affect overall health?

Swami Satyananda: Our body functions along simple lines. Just as a machine produces wastes, the physical body continuously produces wastes. These wastes are of three types: mucus, gas and acidity. If the body is internally cleansed from time to time, the excess of these three metabolic products is removed, and their formation is regulated and balanced. Perfect health can then be maintained.

This is why the practices of the six hatha yoga shatkarmas are of such great importance. Cleansing the body of the three types of wastes accumulated in the system is an important aspect of hatha yoga therapy.

Can concentration be improved by practising the shatkarmas?

Swami Satyananda: When one sits for prayers or pooja, the mind cannot concentrate. Why not? It is true that people with the capacity for real concentration are rare in this world but although the fickleness of the mind is not entirely due to the body, how often is it recognized that the body is partly responsible for the wanderings and waverings of the mind?

To remedy this, make neti a daily practice. Do dhauti frequently at first, then once a week. Practise basti according to any disease requirement. Trataka should be done regularly and kapalbhati does not take much time. Nauli is necessary in basti. Basti is incomplete without nauli. After this, take a glass of water and drink it.

How do shatkarmas prepare the body for advanced practices?

Swami Niranjanananda: Neti, dhauti and basti are the three practices of internal physical purification. Kapalbhati, nauli and trataka are the three practices for mental purification and harmony. The propagators of hatha yoga included trataka in the group of shatkarmas although it is not a physical exercise of purification. It is not like neti, dhauti, basti, kapalbhati or nauli. Trataka is a technique of meditation, yet it is considered to be a cleansing, purifying, relaxing and harmonizing technique due to its immediate effect on the brain and mind.

When these shatkarmas are practised along with the four groups of asanas – pawanmuktasana parts one and two, the shakti bandhas and the trikonasana series – the body is prepared to eventually move on to advanced asanas, which continue to help relieve any diseased condition. Hatha yoga as it is recognized today incorporates shatkarmas, mudras and bandhas, as well as some advanced asanas and pranayamas.

Why are the shatkarmas necessary as preparation for pranayama and meditation?

Swami Satyananda: Pranayama is more effective in a healthy body. If the body is clogged with old mucus, bile and wind, the energy gained through pranayama practice will be used for rectifying those disorders. If one has mucus blockages it can create such an acute problem that pranayama cannot be practised. One must first rid the body of excess mucus and bile and eliminate the toxins from the system. Proper assimilation and excretion have to be established.

The body has three faults: kapha, pitta, and vata. Their imbalance causes disease. In the same way, the mind has three faults. The first one is *mala*, impurity, the second is *vikshepa*, distraction, and the third is *avarana*, ignorance. In *Hatha Yoga Pradipika* (2:36) it is written:

> *Shatkarmanirgatasthaulyakaphadoshamalaadikah.*
> *Praanaayaamam tatah kuryaadanaayaasena siddhyati.*
>
> By the six karmas, (shatkarmas), one is freed from excesses of the doshas. Pranayama can then be practised and success achieved without strain.

Impurity is the psychological stuff which manifests when one sits for meditation. There are five types: *kama*, sensual desire, *krodha*, anger, *moha*, infatuation, *mada*, arrogance or pride, *matsarya*, envy. When visions float across the mind and the mind cannot be made steady due to constant oscillation, that is *vikshepa*. When the mind is unable to understand itself, that is ignorance, *avarana*.

Through the practice of shatkarma the centres in the physical body which are responsible for arousing these doshas in the mind are stabilized. Shatkarma works on the physical body to influence the mind, brainwaves and blockages of energy.

How effective are the shatkarmas at eliminating diseases?

Swami Niranjanananda: Just as simple and dynamic asanas prepare the musculoskeletal system for the advanced therapeutic asanas, the internal organs need energizing and their stamina improving by the practice of shatkarmas. In hatha yoga, the shatkarmas aim at reducing the intensity of mala, vikara and vikshepa.

Mala means an environment or condition which is incompatible with the growth and development of human life. When one lives in that environment for a long time, mala becomes the cause of a disease. Miners who work in coal mines hundreds of metres underground continuously inhale different kinds of gases and coal dust for eight hours a day. These people often suffer from tuberculosis, asthma and respiratory problems due to the effect of the detrimental environment on the body.

There are people who drink impure water containing thousands of bacteria known and unknown to science. There are water-borne diseases which affect the digestive system, pancreas, liver and kidneys. There are air-borne diseases affecting the lungs. There are chemical-borne diseases affecting the immune system. Scientists have recently found fifty new viruses which are carried by mosquitoes. They can kill, cause cerebral fever or carry other diseases for which there is no antidote. All are classified as mala, impurity.

Vikshepa refers to the mind which is disturbed, unbalanced and confused. Vikshepa always begins as worry or *chintan*, brooding over something. When vikshepa begins, it changes the state of mind. A dynamic mind can become lethargic, a clear mind can become confused, a positive mind can become negative. This change of the mental state affects the nervous system. When a dynamic mind becomes lethargic, it changes the whole physical system and increases the parasympathetic activity, thus lowering the normal vitality and immunity of the body.

Genetically everyone is born with one weaker organ. In some people the lungs may be weak, in some people the heart, in some the muscles, in some the bones, in others the liver or the kidneys. Everybody has what is known as their

Achilles heel. Vikshepa affects that weak organ. If the lungs are weak and one is passing through the state of vikshepa, breathlessness will manifest. If the digestion is weak and one is going through vikshepa, diarrhoea and dysentery will manifest. If the liver is weak, liver-related problems will manifest. If the joints are weak, one will suddenly become aware of pains which were not there before. Vikshepa will always attack the weakest organ of the body and the problem will start increasing from that point onwards.

Vikara means toxins. Even in a healthy life, toxins accumulate in the body. Accumulated toxins are normally excreted in sweat, urine and faeces, but sometimes the excretion is less than the amount that has been taken in. The toxins then go into the blood and are absorbed by the body, for example, into the muscles. They also become part of the natural acids of the body, such as lactic acid. One can be a healthy and dynamic person, but if there is a build up of toxins in the body, whenever there is a period of inactivity in one's life, the toxins and acids begin to build up in various joints, and if one stretches, there is a feeling of stiffness. This stiffness can become pain, and the pain can become arthritis. The build up of acids and toxins can deform the bones, making them brittle, as happens in osteoporosis.

It can be said that vikara involves the somatic group of illnesses, vikshepa involves the psychosomatic group of illnesses and mala involves the environmental pollutants and unhygienic conditions which cause illness.

While preparing the body for advanced practices, another miracle happens. As one reduces vikara and mala in one's personality and nature, many of the physical, psychosomatic or spiritual problems are automatically reduced. Disease and illness, whether physical, mental or spiritual, are generated when there is an accumulation of toxins. It is like saying, 'Mosquitoes do not breed in flowing water, they only breed in stagnant water.' If the energy is flowing and the body is pure, there is little chance for the roots of disease to go into the body and personality.

Therefore, people often begin to feel better without actually using any major postures for therapy, but just with the practice of pawanmuktasana and shatkarmas.

It is the experience of many yoga teachers that about forty to fifty percent of problems, diseases and illnesses are helped with only the basic group of shatkarmas and pawanmuktasana. The people who are not helped by these basic practices are helped once they move on to advanced asanas. Therefore, the practice of basic yoga is always emphasized rather than advanced yoga practices. Advanced yoga is taught when necessary, but the practice of pawanmuktasana is always recommended and emphasized. If one can practise neti, kunjal and laghoo shankhaprakshalana in its most basic form, up to forty to fifty percent of one's health will be regained. Whatever is not regained by this method will be regained with the help of advanced asanas, which directly affect the internal organs of the body.

Does purification of the body through shatkarmas lengthen the lifespan?

Swami Niranjanananda: After purification a human being lives longer on this earth. The Upanishads and Vedas state in a number of places that human beings live for a hundred years. This is not only the thinking of the Vedas, Upanishads or ancient philosophies, it is the truth. If a human being remains healthy and free from disease, living for a hundred years or more is natural. Accurate genetic copying of the cells can continue for that length of time if the programming is not disrupted by impurities or imbalances.

SHATKARMAS AND THE PRANAMAYA KOSHA

How does purifying the physical body affect the pranic body?

Swami Satyananda: It is said in hatha yoga that in this physical body there are hundreds and thousands of channels or flows of energy, and everywhere this energy is facing a blockage due to impurities. What is hatha yoga? Nowadays people think that postures are hatha yoga, but actually hatha yoga is a systematic practice in which the purification of the physical body is taught.

There are six practices through which the physical body is purified. When the body is purified, these nadis or channels of energy become free of obstruction and the pranas flow freely, the consciousness flows freely. There is no blockage; one can experience perfect health, a perfect state of mind, and perfect understanding of one's self.

Is it necessary to practise the shatkarmas in preparation for pranayama?

Swami Sivananda: Those who are of a flabby and phlegmatic constitution should practise the shatkarmas as preparation for pranayama. Success will then come easily.

What is the main purpose of the shatkarmas?

Swami Satyananda: The purpose of emphasizing the shatkarmas is to prepare a base for higher pranayama. The shatkarmas purify the whole system and remove the blockages on the paths of prana, *pingala nadi*, and the mind, *ida nadi*. When there are no blockages on the pathways of ida and pingala, the breath in both nostrils flows systematically.

What are the most important practices for purifying the nadis?

Swami Satyananda: Before the awakening of chakras, before purification of the chakras, before checking the functioning order of the chakras, one must purify the nadis. Purification of nadis is known as *nadi shodhana* or *nadi shuddhi*; purification of the chakras is *chakra shodhana*, *chakra shuddhi*.

There are two important yogic practices for the purification of the nadis. One is known as shatkarma and the other as pranayama. Through the practice of the shatkarmas, the material aspect of the nadi is purified, through the practice of pranayama, the energy aspect of the nadi is purified, and both have to be taken care of.

How do the shatkarmas affect the five koshas of the body?

Swami Satyananda: When the body is purified, the chemical constituents are in balanced proportion and the brain functions are simultaneously influenced and altered. When the body is pure the mind becomes stable, emotional reactions to external stimuli are altered and one responds in a more relaxed and controlled manner. Therefore, shatkarmas bring control over unruly senses. They make the *karmendriya*, organs of action, keen, and the *jnanendriya*, organs of knowledge, more perceptive and sensitive. The shatkarmas not only purify the body elements or *dhatu*, they also influence the subtle body.

According to yoga, human existence extends through five layers or sheaths which are called *koshas*. The physical body and its elements comprise the first layer, *annamaya kosha*.

Anna is 'food', *maya* means 'comprised of'. The shatkarmas directly influence this kosha and penetrate the next layer, *pranamaya kosha*, the energy body, by allowing free flow of prana in the physical body. The third layer, *manomaya kosha*, the mental sheath, is indirectly affected through pranayama. Purification of these sheaths opens the fourth kosha, *vijnanamaya* or the sheath of intuition. However, the fifth kosha, *anandamaya* or the sheath of bliss, is unaffected by any physical influence as it is a transcendental realm.

These five sheaths are interlinked; whatever happens in one affects the others. When annamaya and pranamaya are cleansed there are no blockages between them and manomaya. Mind, body and energy can work in unison, removing the barrier to vijnanamaya kosha.

The first four koshas are extensions of anandamaya. When there are blockages between any of the koshas, communication and integration are hindered. Annamaya and pranamaya are gross manifestations while manomaya and vijnanamaya are subtle. Pranamaya is the link between the gross and subtle and manomaya is the bridge to the higher mind. When one practises the shatkarmas, integration of the whole being is established, physically, emotionally, mentally, psychically and cosmically.

How does one know which shatkarmas to practise for balancing the nadis?

Swami Satyananda: With the guidance of an experienced teacher, the shatkarmas are done according to one's requirements and capacity. After practising these shatkarmas for one to two years, harmony is attained within the parasympathetic and sympathetic nervous systems, and in ida and pingala nadis, which are responsible for *manas shakti*, mental energy and *prana shakti*, pranic or vital energy. If either of these nadis are disturbed, diseases born of manas or prana shakti develop.

How do wastes in the physical body interfere with the pranic body?

Swami Satyananda: The interior of the body must be pure. For example, fermentation of mucus interferes with the pranic activities. That is why the stomach, intestines, nose, mouth and whole body must be properly cleaned. This physical body is a combination and permutation of the five elements: ether, air, fire, water and earth. If these five elements are not purified, they interfere with the activities of prana. In order to purify these elements in the body, hatha yoga must be practised.

Is purification of the body necessary before the awakening of kundalini?

Swami Sivananda: Rousing of kundalini and its union with Shiva at sahasrara chakra bring about the states of samadhi and mukti. Before awakening the kundalini, one must have purity of body, purification of nadis, purity of mind and purity of intellect. For the purification of the body, the hatha yoga shatkarmas are prescribed.

Is it possible to awaken the chakras by practising only the shatkarmas?

Swami Niranjanananda: The chakras are not situated in the mental body, nor are they situated in the physical body, although they are represented in them. They are actually situated in the causal body. The awakening of the chakras takes place on all levels: the body, the mind, and the causal levels. Just through the practices of the hatha yoga shatkarmas, it is possible to awaken all the chakras without the need of practising asanas or any form of pranayama. It is also possible to awaken kundalini through these practices alone. In *Hatharatnavali* (1:59) it is written:

> *Shatchakrashodhanam samyak praanaayaamasya kaaranam.*
> *Naashanam sarvarogaanaam mokshamaargasya saadhanam.*
>
> These eight purificatory processes purify the six chakras thoroughly and all types of diseases are destroyed. It is the way to attain moksha and also the base for practising pranayama.

Hatharatnavali (1:61–66) then gives details of the effects on the various chakras:

> *Aadhaarashodhanam chakryaa lingam vajrolikarmanaa.*
>
> *Manipooram naabhigatam naulyaakhyena tu karmanaa.*
>
> *Hridayam kanthachakrastham dhautyaakhyena tu karmanaa.*
>
> *Shodhanam kaaryamaajnaayaam netitrotana karmanaa.*
>
> *Sarvaangashodhanam kaaryam vasti bhastrika karmanaa.*
> *Syaadaadhaaram svaadhishthaanam manipooramanaahatam.*
>
> *Vishuddham kanthachakrastham ajnaachakram bhruvormukhe.*
> *Chakrabhedamitijnaatvaa chakraateeta niranjanam.*
>
> The base is purified through chakri karma and the male organ is purified through vajroli karma. (61)

Manipura, situated in the navel region, is purified through the karma named nauli. (62)

The chakra situated in the region of the heart and throat is purified through the karma named dhauti. (63)

Purification of ajna chakra is done through neti and trataka karmas. (64)

One should purify the whole body through basti and bhastrika process. These chakras are mooladhara, swadhisthana, manipura, and anahata. (65)

Vishuddhi chakra is situated in the throat and ajna chakra is situated in the middle of the eyebrows. In this way after knowing the different chakras, one should know the niranjana (stainless) state which is beyond chakra. (66)

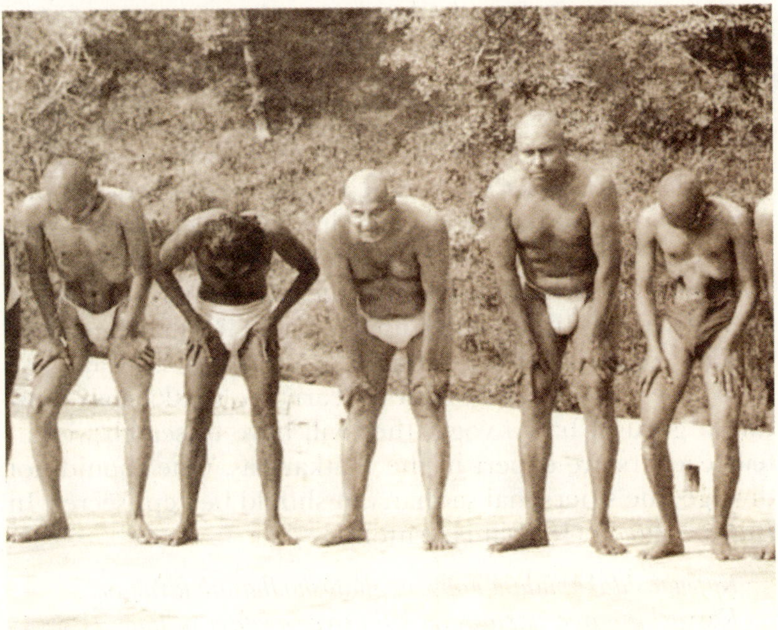

2

Shatkarma Sadhana

GENERAL GUIDELINES

What is the ideal environment for practising the shatkarmas?

Swami Sivananda: The place of practice should be carefully chosen. Practise in seclusion, alone in a room with no object nearby, just as one does for asana practice.

How should one learn the shatkarmas?

Swami Satyananda: The shatkarmas are said to be secret practices. These powerful techniques should never be learned from books or taught by inexperienced people. According to the tradition, only those instructed by a guru may teach others. It is essential to be personally instructed as to how and when to perform the shatkarmas, according to individual limitations and needs. A qualified and experienced teacher is essential.

Those who sincerely want to learn the shatkarmas must find a guru of hatha yoga: they will have to search well as few teachers are expert in the shatkarmas. One should not divulge one's personal sadhana, it should be kept secret. In *Hatharatnavali* (1:27) it is written:

Karmaashtakamidam gopyam ghatashodhanakaarakam.
Kasyachinnaiva vaktavyam kulastree suratam yathaa.

These eight purificatory processes are most secret and they purify the body. One should not talk about them to anyone as a respectable woman does not talk about her sexual enjoyment.

Should all sadhakas practise shatkarmas to balance the doshas?

Swami Satyananda: There are three *doshas*, or humours in the body: *kapha*, mucus, *pitta*, bile and *vata*, wind. In yoga and ayurveda they are called *tridosha*. A balanced proportion of these three facilitates bodily functions, but if there is an excess of one and a shortage of another, ailments develop due to overheating or not enough heat in the body.

Before commencing pranayama, any imbalance in the doshas should be removed – excess body fat should be reduced, mucus blocking the respiratory tract should be removed and gas in the stomach and intestines eliminated. In *Hatha Yoga Pradipika* (2:21) it states:

> *Medashleshmaadhikah poorvam shatkarmaani samaacharet.*
> *Anyastu naacharettaani doshaanaam samabhaavatah.*
>
> When fat or mucus is excessive, shatkarma, the six cleansing techniques, should be practised before (pranayama). Others, in whom the doshas, i.e. phlegm, wind and bile, are balanced, should not do them.

If the doshas are already balanced there is no need to practise the shatkarmas. They should be learned, however, so that the sadhaka will know how to practise them if they are needed. If they are practised unnecessarily, as a part of one's daily sadhana, they will not be so effective when genuinely required. Just as one would not have one's tonsils or appendix removed if they were functioning perfectly, similarly, the shatkarmas are really only for those people who have disturbances or imbalances in the doshas.

Why is it necessary to change one's lifestyle when taking up hatha yoga?

Swami Satyananda: Practices such as shankhaprakshalana exert a profound cleansing and purifying effect upon the subtle body, and demand dietary regulation if the states of awareness generated are to be preserved and consolidated. What is the point in doing shankhaprakshalana if after a week one again begins to eat greasy and tamasic foods, starts smoking and so on? Unhealthy habits only maintain blockages in the nadis.

The practices of hatha yoga are powerful, and they demand responsibility and self-discipline. Otherwise, it is not only a waste of time, but also foolhardy and dangerous. Therefore, along with the initial practices of hatha yoga, a conducive lifestyle must gradually emerge.

Are there any restrictions on women practising the shatkarmas during menstruation?

Swami Niranjanananda: There are no absolute restrictions and rules for the practices of neti, trataka or kapalbhati, but during the practices of dhauti, basti and nauli, one should ensure that no undue pressure is created in the sensitive female system at the time of the monthly cycle. If undue pressure and tension is created in the muscular structure the hormonal cycle can be affected. Therefore, the practices of neti, kapalbhati and trataka can be practised during menstruation, while those of dhauti, basti and nauli are better done afterwards to avoid any kind of hormonal or glandular imbalance within the body.

What diet should be followed during the practice of shatkarma?

Swami Satyananda: In regard to diet, there are different opinions. Some authorities recommend a lot of fat, milk, fruits and vegetables. This is an aristocratic point of view. Others believe in a socialist diet, which means whole wheat, unpolished rice boiled in water which remains in the rice, green peas, corn, unpeeled potatoes, etc. Germinated beans and wheat are recommended. Yogic texts state that the food should not be over-spiced, over-boiled, over-tasty or over-fried.

All fresh foods are recommended, except meat, fish and eggs. There are scientific as well as religious reasons why animal products are not taken. Meat contains poison produced by the animal's body at the time of killing. Also, meat decomposes fast and creates toxicity in the system. Digestion of meat, as with any food rich in protein but poor in acid, demands high secretions of digestive juices, which the alimentary system cannot produce. Therefore, alcohol is often used to help the digestive process. Some fish contain an oil which may cause allergic conditions. Eggs destroy the structure of the kidneys and cause albumen secretion in the urinary system, so the long term effects are not beneficial.

Srikhand is the usual meal of hatha yogis. The water is removed from curd which is hung in cloth in a warm room for several days. Cardamom, saffron and other ingredients are then added and the mixture is churned for several hours, producing a sattwic meal. Diet is generally only discussed in reference to hatha yoga, however, diet should not only be adjusted by hatha yoga practitioners. For raja, karma and bhakti yoga the diet is also important.

SEQUENCE AND TIMING

What is the correct sequence for practising shatkarmas?

Swami Satyananda: When integral yoga is practised with an emphasis on hatha yoga, practise of the shatkarmas is in the following order:

1. Practise dhauti before going to the toilet after rising in the morning.
2. Practise neti during the morning bath.
3. Practise nauli after neti and asanas, but before pranayama and meditation.
4. Practise kapalbhati after pranayama, on an empty stomach.

5. Practise trataka after asanas and pranayama, but before meditation and yoga nidra. During the hot season trataka should only be done in the morning. In winter trataka can also be done at night.

Basti should only be practised to remove constipation. In that case, practise before taking a bath.

What is the best season for the practice of the shatkarmas?

Swami Satyananda: Spring is the best time to start the practice of hatha yoga. In India, this is during the month of March, when the weather is neither too cold nor too hot, there is little difference in the temperature between day and night, and there is a balanced temperature of body and atmosphere.

Should the shatkarmas be practised when one starts learning hatha yoga?

Swami Satyananda: Sometimes the shatkarmas should be taught before asana and pranayama, and sometimes they can be taught simultaneously. If the student is very weak, they should be taught later. The practice of neti can be taught at any time. The practices of kunjal and shankhaprakshalana should be taught later, after some time. The teacher must think about the student's capacity.

Should shatkarmas be practised before pranayama?

Swami Satyananda: There are two differing opinions about the necessity of practising the shatkarmas prior to pranayama. Some hatha yoga teachers say that one should first clean the nadis through shatkarmas so that pranayama will be effective. Others believe that pranayama alone will remove the blockages in the nadis and balance all elements of the body. Both opinions are correct, but which to follow? In *Hatha Yoga Pradipika* (2:37) it says:

Praanaayaamaireva sarve prashushyanti malaa iti.
Aachaaryaanaam tu keshaanchidanyatkarma na sammatam.

According to some teachers, pranayama alone removes impurities and therefore they hold pranayama in esteem and not the other techniques.

Shatkarmas provide a quick method of rebalancing mucus, bile and wind. If the body is first cleansed through shatkarma, pranayama will maintain that state of cleanliness. If one has excess mucus, bile or wind and practises pranayama only, the energy generated through pranayama will all be spent in rectifying the state of imbalance. If, however, the body is healthy, the nadis are clean and the whole system is functioning in harmony, pranayama can be practised without any need for shatkarma. If there is a slight imbalance, pranayama alone will be sufficient to rectify any problem.

Excess mucus is the major obstacle which prevents pranayama practice. When the nose or respiratory tract is completely blocked, pranayama is impossible, so one will definitely have to resort to neti, kunjal or even laghoo shankhaprakshalana. For nasal congestion, neti and kunjal are sufficient, but for respiratory congestion, asthma or bronchitis, the three karmas will be necessary. In *Hatharatnavali* (1:58) it is written:

Karmaashtabhirgatasthaulyam kaphamedo malaadhikah.
Praanaayaamam tatah kuryaadanaayaasena sidhyati.

The aspirant should do pranayama after getting rid of corpulence, phlegm, fat and other impurities by means of the eight purificatory processes. Then he will succeed in yoga without much difficulty.

Although the shatkarmas are powerful and effective purifiers and harmonizers, pranayama has to be practised afterwards to maintain the balance they have created. Otherwise impurities will again accumulate and the body will fall back into its old patterns.

What is the best system for practising the shatkarmas?

Swami Niranjanananda: There has to be a proper system for practising the hatha yoga shatkarmas. Begin with neti as it helps to clear the nasal passages of mucus blocks, allowing for proper intake of air through the nostrils. Neti not only allows optimum breathing, but also aids in relaxing and sensitizing the nervous system, an effect which is beneficial in the advanced practices of hatha yoga and other yogas.

After neti, kapalbhati should be performed. This helps one develop greater control over the autonomic muscular movements of the body. Control over the diaphragm, abdominal muscles, lungs, chest, and the muscles surrounding the lungs, chest and ribcage, are attained through the practice of kapalbhati. In this way, the muscles are gradually trained for other practices.

Mental relaxation is as important as physical relaxation at the time of yoga sadhana. For this, trataka can be practised to release tensions from the mind, intellect and emotions. The resulting tranquillity, starting with the inner personality, influences the physical body.

Next, the practice of nauli should be done. Nauli gives control over the movement of the small and subtle muscles of the internal system.

After nauli, different forms of dhauti should be performed to prepare the system gradually for the final practice of basti.

Basti should be practised last, as in basti the natural laws of the body are reversed. The natural process is to expel bodily waste through the anus and urinary tracts. However, by taking in air, water or other forms of liquid through the anus, the nature of the pranic flow and of the muscular structure are reversed, requiring a great deal of control of the nerves, muscles and organs. Therefore, basti should be practised last.

How can shatkarma practise be fitted into a busy lifestyle?

Swami Niranjanananda: Shatkarmas can be done on the weekends to remove the impurities and toxins that have accumulated in the body during the week. On Sunday, drop the morning practice of asana and pranayama and instead do one shatkarma, such as neti, kunjal, or laghoo shankhaprakshalana.

Kunjal – drinking water and regurgitating it – helps maintain an active digestive system and remove toxins such as bile, acidity, wind, gasses and mucus from the digestive system. Once a week, to detoxify, the stomach and oesophagus should be cleaned with kunjal. It needs to be learnt under proper guidance so that the teacher can decide whether it is a suitable practice or not.

Neti – nasal cleaning – is practiced after kunjal. It can be done by everyone. It is good for migraine, good for improving short-sightedness, and good for improving the auditory system. Neti is also good for the brain, eyes, ears, nose and throat. Once a week this cleaning should take place. Many pollutants are breathed in all day, accumulating in the sinuses. Due to this, allergies develop and the sinuses become inflamed. Weather affects the sinuses, inflamed sinuses affect the eyesight and the frontal region of the brain. They can also cause headaches. Therefore, to maintain the health of the face and head, practise neti once a week.

3

Neti: Nasal Cleansing

WHAT IS NETI?

Why is it important to keep the nostrils clean?

Swami Sivananda: Neti is for the purification of the nostrils. The nostrils must always be kept clean. Unclean nostrils lead to irregular breathing, and irregular breathing makes one sick. Head colds and hay fever are cured with neti. In *Gheranda Samhita* (1:51) it is stated that neti kriya produces *divya drishti*, clairvoyance:

> *Saadhanaannetikaaryasya khechareesiddhimaapnuyaat;*
> *Kaphadoshaa vinashyanti divyadrishtih prajaayate.*
>
> The practice of neti enables one to attain perfection in khechari, elimination of kapha and attainment of divine vision.

What is neti?

Swami Satyananda: Neti is the kriya of cleansing the eyes, nose and throat with water, milk, urine or a catheter through the nose. These centres and senses are cleaned and made free from impurities. It is the first shatkarma of hatha yoga.

Most commonly, warm saline water is passed through one nostril and comes out the other. If there is any nasal blockage a catheter which enters through the nostril and comes out through the mouth, is used. It is a practice designed to clean the nasal passages, reduce the amount of waste material deposited there and allow a greater amount of oxygen to pass into the brain. Neti cures infections, colds, cataracts, sinusitis, migraine, infection of the adenoids, polyps and inflammation of the nasal membrane.

Neti also activates the brain: neti is the cleaning of the nasal passage in order to awaken sushumna.

Why is neti the first shatkarma practice in hatha yoga?

Swami Niranjanananda: The first cleansing technique of hatha yoga is neti, which translates simply as nasal cleaning. Neti originated, however, not as a practice of nasal cleaning, but as a technique for awakening the centres related to ajna chakra. When the sinuses are blocked, one can feel the tension near the eyes and forehead, where the pressure and blockages are experienced. Due to blocked sinuses, one may have watering and reddening of the eyes, and ear blockages. Yogis considered this part of the head to be extremely sensitive, so they put cleaning of the general nasal area, which affects the eyes and ears, first.

How was neti traditionally practised?

Swami Niranjanananda: Two forms of neti are commonly known: *jala neti*, in which warm saline water is used, and *sutra neti*, in which a catheter is used to clean the nasal passages.

The original form of jala neti involved drinking a glass of cold water through the nose and expelling it through the mouth. This was a common practice in Indian villages, called *ushapaan*. Every morning after brushing their teeth, the elders of the family would drink a glass of water through their nose.

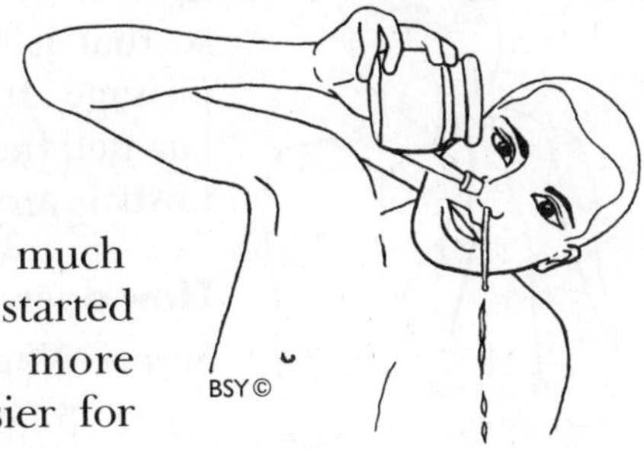

The neti *lota*, or pot, came much later when Swami Satyananda started making the yogic practices more accessible, acceptable and easier for all. Neti becomes a simple process with a neti lota. The spout is simply put into one nostril to pour the water, which then flows out through the other nostril.

What is the practice of nasal cleansing with thread?

Swami Satyananda: The practice of passing a length of thread through the nose is called *sutra neti*. *Sutra* means, thread. This is described in *Hatha Yoga Pradipika* (2:29):

> *Sootram vitastisusnigdham naasaanaale praveshayet.*
> *Mukhaannirgamayechchaishaa netih siddhairnigadyate.*
>
> Insert a soft thread through the nose to the length of one handspan so that it comes out of the mouth. This is called neti by the siddhas.

To practise sutra neti a specially prepared thread has to be used. It should be made of cotton, not synthetic fibre, tightly wound together and wiped with melted beeswax. The width should be about 4 mm, and the length, 36 cm. In *Hatharatnavali* (1:37) it is written:

> *Atha neti karma*
> *Aakhupuchchhaakaaranibham sootram susnigdhanirmitam.*
> *Shadvitastimitam sootram netisootrasya lakshanam.*
>
> A smooth thread made like the tail of the rat, and of four and a half feet in length is the neti thread.

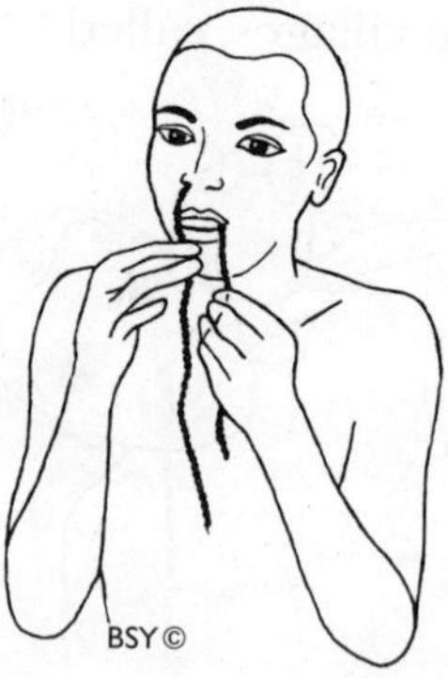

However, it is more convenient to use a thin rubber catheter lubricated with ghee so that it slides easily through the nasal passage. It is also a good idea to practise jala neti before sutra neti to make sure the nostrils are clear.

How does neti work?

Swami Niranjanananda: When lukewarm water passes through the nostrils, its influence is first felt by the tissue lining the nose and sinuses. Glands within this tissue produce mucus which traps germs and other particles. This tissue also regulates the temperature of air inside the nose before it passes into the lungs. When air is cold it is brought nearer to body temperature before passing inside. The nose acts like a strainer and air passes through its holes. Sometimes when the nose becomes stuffy, one cannot breathe properly as all the pores of the strainer are blocked, and the nose's air conditioning effect is lost.

Air passing through the nose also travels into the sinuses. Sinuses are cavities within the bones of the face and skull, similar to the cavities that are observed in a sponge. Sinuses are situated in the area around the eyebrow centre. There are many subtle nadis in this region, which are connected to the sinuses. Of these, some nadis are related to the eyes and some to the ears, while others go inside the brain.

Breathing is a process which people are not generally concerned about, even though it continues uninterrupted throughout one's life; it goes on unknowingly. Even when one sleeps at night, the breathing continues. A person becomes aware of the nose only when mucus collects or increases in the eyebrow centre region, or when there is congestion in the sinuses. Then one thinks, "I have a nose I have to be careful with."

Often mucus inside the nose becomes dry during summer. Irritation is then felt due to the hot air. Often when the nose is blocked, there is also a feeling of heaviness in the eyes. The ears might feel somewhat blocked as well, and there is a feeling of heaviness in the brain. Generally when mucus inside becomes dry, one blows it out. Dust particles which are caught in the mucus are also expelled. If one is in a place where the environment is dirty, polluted and impure, there may often be a feeling of heaviness in the head, or a headache. The eyes also become red and start watering, and with only a little reading, become irritated and painful. Heaviness of the eyes, ears and head is not only linked with the outside heat, but also with the warmth of the breath. If neti is performed, there is immediate relief.

Suppose one is near a coal mine, where coal dust abounds; when the nose is blown, black mucus comes out. Coal dust is found in the lungs of workers employed in coal mines; people working in such an environment are prone to respiratory disorders. All the impurities cannot be expelled by simply blowing the nose. Dry and sticky particles are left, which is why the practice of neti is essential in such circumstances.

During neti, when the water enters one nostril and comes out through the other, a number of processes simultaneously take place. The most obvious is the expulsion of waste products and mucus with the flow of water through the other nostril. When people with colds practise neti, not much water comes out at first. Mucus comes out with a few drops of water. The mucus is gradually loosened, and slowly comes out. The mucous membrane, through which air enters, is cleaned in this way.

A more subtle effect is that when water enters and passes through the nostrils and eyebrow centre region, mild sensations are created in all the nadis of that area. Neti has a beneficial influence on the subtle nadis and nerves of the nose, which are connected to the nadis of the eyes and ears. If there is any disorder pertaining to the eyes or ears, the practice of neti is helpful. Sometimes tears may flow when practising neti, but they do not cause any discomfort or burning sensation. Neti stimulates the nerves around the eyes, and due to this they start watering.

NETI TECHNIQUES

What are the different types of neti and how are they practised?

Swami Satyananda: There are six techniques for cleaning the nasal passages:

1. *Jala neti*: Luke warm, saline water is either sucked or poured through one nostril and allowed to come out of the

other. While practising, the breath is suspended and the mouth is open. The same process is repeated with the other nostril.

A small pot with a spout can be used to pour the water through one nostril and out the other, while breathing through the open mouth. This is the easiest method for beginners.

2. *Sutra neti*: Either a rubber catheter or a thick cotton thread is inserted gently through one nostril and brought out through the mouth or the other nostril. Holding both ends of the catheter, it is pulled to and fro to stimulate the nasal orifice. The same process is repeated through the other nostril. This should be followed by *dugdha*, milk, neti. Sutra neti is beneficial if there is a deviated septum or chronic nasal blockage which water cannot pass. In *Hatharatvavali* (1:38–39) sutra neti is described:

> *Naasaanaale praveshyainam mukhaannirgamayetkramaat.*
> *Sootrasyaantam prabaddhvaa tu bhraamayennaasanaalayoh.*
>
> *Manthanam cha tatah kuryaannetih siddhairnigadyate.*
>
> Introducing it in one nostril, it should be taken out from the mouth gradually. By joining the two ends of the thread, it should be rotated through the nostrils. (38)
>
> Then one should churn it through (the nostrils), this is called neti by the siddhas. (39)

3. *Dugdha neti*: Using milk which has been boiled and strained, the same procedure is followed as for jala neti. This practice is not generally done independently, but as a follow up to sutra neti. Dugdha neti is essential for pranayama when the nasal passages are too dry. It is beneficial for problems of the eyes and throat. It also cures vertigo when it is due to nasal infections.

4. *Ghrita neti*: Using melted ghee, the same procedure as for jala neti is followed.

5. *Tel neti*: Using pure mustard oil which has been slightly burned, the same instructions as for jala neti are followed.

6. *Bhastrika neti*: Breathing rapidly through the right and left nostrils independently and then through both nostrils together, this practice is done at the end of all the five netis in order to dry the nasal passages.

What equipment is needed for jala neti?

Swami Satyananda: A pot or lota is used to pour salt water into the nostrils. There are various designs and even a teapot can be used if nothing else is available. This pot is known as a *neti lota*. It can be made of brass, stainless steel, plastic or any other suitable material which does not contaminate water. The important point to remember is that the nozzle on the end of the spout should be suitably sized so that the end fits comfortably into the nostril.

Why is salt water used in jala neti?

Swami Satyananda: People often wonder why salt water is introduced into the nostrils instead of ordinary water. The reason is simple and practical. Salt water has a much higher osmotic pressure than ordinary water, which means that salt water is not easily absorbed into the delicate blood vessels and membranes in the nose, whereas ordinary water is. If this practice is tried with ordinary water it causes discomfort or a little pain in the nose. Salt water is ideal for jala neti, as it thoroughly cleans the nostrils of impurities but is not absorbed into the delicate nasal membranes. This means that no discomfort is felt when the water flows through the nose.

Why is amaroli used for neti?

Swami Niranjanananda: Amaroli neti uses the midstream of the first urination for the day. The amaroli is collected in a pot and one or two drops are added to pure water. Neti is then performed with this solution. Urine is acidic and is an excellent anti-infection agent. Uric acid destroys germs, thus helping to eradicate many disorders. Some people use their undiluted urine in neti for therapeutic purposes. This has a subtle drying effect on delicate tissue, so if neti is done with undiluted urine it should be followed with salt water neti after five or ten minutes.

What other liquids can be used for neti?

Swami Niranjanananda: Other than salt water, hatha yoga practitioners also use other liquids, including warm milk or ghee to perfect neti. First the nostrils are washed with jala neti, then neti is performed using milk or ghee or any other natural edible oil. The practice is done by sniffing a small amount of the fluid into the nose from a glass or bowl. Groundnut oil or olive oil can also be used. Mustard oil gives a burning sensation, but some people use it. Sesame oil is also used. Neti kriya includes all these practices.

How is the thread made for sutra neti?

Swami Satyananda: One has to know how to make the thread. In India two or three cotton threads are twisted together, then soaked in wax to make it stiff. But in the west the wax is not pure, and no-one knows what chemicals have been added. Therefore it is safer to use a rubber catheter.

How does the practice of neti change as one becomes more experienced?

Swami Niranjanananda: As one becomes more experienced, the viscosity of the liquid used to clean the nostrils can be increased. For example, some hatha yogis practise neti with oil, ghee, milk and even yoghurt. Each practice gives a different benefit. If oil is used, the effect will be different to using water. If amaroli is used, the result is different to using milk. It has been said that once the sinus passages are cleared and optimum functioning of the optical and auditory nerves is achieved, ajna chakra can be activated.

GUIDELINES FOR PRACTICE

Why should neti be practised even when the nose is not blocked?

Swami Satyananda: Regular practice of neti when one doesn't have a cold keeps the nasal passages working at optimum efficiency and thereby helps maintain a healthy body. Remember, breathing through the mouth or insufficient treatment of the inhaled air prior to entry into the lungs, due to nasal blockage and congestion, can encourage the onset of disease by allowing germs to infect the lungs, or by generally weakening the body.

How long does it take to practise neti and when is the ideal time?

Swami Satyananda: Once the practitioner is familiar with the technique, the whole practice can be completed in a short period of time. Not including preparation of the water, the whole process should take less than five minutes.

Neti is ideally practised early in the morning before breakfast. If necessary, however, it can be practised at other times of the day, excepting straight after meals.

How often should neti be practised?

Swami Satyananda: Initially jala neti can be done every day and those who suffer from excess mucus can continue to practise daily. Those who suffer from sinusitis, colds, insensitivity to smell, headache, eyestrain or eye infections, can practise daily, otherwise only once or twice a week is necessary. If one has nasal catarrh, a cold or any other specific ailment, neti may be practised more than once a day.

When should neti be avoided?

Swami Satyananda: Neti should not be practised directly after eating or drinking. It should not be done if there are any perforations in the walls of the nasal passages due to high blood pressure. People suffering from chronic nosebleed should not attempt neti unless under expert guidance.

What precautions are there for the practice of neti?

Swami Niranjanananda: Ensure that the water used is not too hot. While drying the nostrils, do not blow out of the nose with excessive force. Before commencing the practice it is important to ensure that the salt is properly dissolved.

If there is persistent difficulty getting water to flow through the nostrils, there may be some obstruction within the nose. In such cases, an expert should be consulted. Do not worry if there is initially a little irritation while passing water through the nostrils; as one becomes accustomed to the practice, irritation will cease.

What is the best posture for practising jala neti?

Swami Satyananda: One may either sit in a squatting position or assume a standing position, bending the shoulders and head forwards. The standing position is most suitable for doing neti into a sink or wash basin, while the squatting position can be done in the garden or in a shower.

Why is the position of the head important when practising neti?

Swami Satyananda: Be careful to hold the head correctly and not to hold the neti pot too low. In order for the water to flow into one nostril and out the other, the water level in the pot must be higher than the region at the back of the nose, where the two nostrils merge with each other. If the head is tilted back too much, the water goes down the throat instead of out the other nostril. If the pot is tilted too much the water will overflow out of the pot. The position of the head and the pot must be adjusted so that they are at correct levels.

What should be done if the water won't flow through the nose?

Swami Satyananda: People who have great difficulty passing water through the nose may have a structural blockage such as a polyp. Expert advice should be sought.

If there is no structural blockage, yet one of the nostrils does not cooperate, try sutra neti, with a thread. Insert the thread and take it out the other nostril. Or, practise bhastrika for ten minutes and the nose should clear. Try different methods and have two-way traffic; in life it is not good to have one-way traffic.

Which nostril is the water poured through first when practising neti?

Swami Niranjanananda: Although some traditionalists hold the view that neti should always begin with the left nostril, and some hold the view that it should begin with the right nostril, it has been our experience that the performance of neti can and should be done with whichever nostril is flowing at the time of practice. This facilitates the entry of water and removes any blockages.

When neti is performed through a blocked nostril, the water won't enter; if it does enter, it is in drops or maybe a trickle. This becomes a time-consuming process. However, the nostril which is open provides an easier entry for the water within the nasal passage, and that water, once it enters, is able to flow out through the other nostril much more easily.

How should beginners develop the practice of sutra neti?

Swami Niranjanananda: In the beginning there will be some difficulty in pulling the thread in and out, as it takes time for the nadis, nerves and mucous membranes to become strong. The practice must be developed gradually, without using undue force. As the nadis become stronger, their efficacy increases. The sutra should be pulled back and forth a maximum of fourteen times. Sutra neti should be done once a week, not daily. The ideal time for its practice is in the morning before breakfast.

Why are other forms of neti practised after sutra neti?

Swami Satyananda: After completing sutra neti one should do jala neti, as this flushes out all the impurities and particles in the nose, including those that have been dislodged by performing sutra neti, leaving the nasal passages in the cleanest possible condition.

After performing both sutra and jala neti, the nasal passages may feel a little sore and raw, and perhaps overly dry. For this reason, the practice should be completed by doing either milk or ghee neti. These are simple techniques which merely involve introducing a few drops of milk or ghee (clarified butter) into the nasal passages. To do this, the head is held back and the fluid sniffed into the nose from a suitable vessel. Only a small amount of milk or ghee is required; don't flood the nose.

Ghee or milk neti temporarily replace the natural protective film of mucus in the nose that has been rubbed or washed away by sutra and jala neti. However, this practice is optional, for the body will manufacture a new film within a short period of time.

If the nostrils are particularly blocked prior to attempting sutra neti, then jala neti can be performed before sutra neti as well as afterwards.

How are the nostrils dried after jala neti?

Swami Satyananda: It is advisable to practise bhastrika or kapalbhati pranayama after jala neti. This will dry the nose and generate heat in the nostrils.

BENEFITS

What are the benefits associated with the various neti techniques?

Swami Satyananda: Sutra neti, which is practised by passing a rubber catheter in the nostril and out of the mouth, is useful for removing most blocked conditions. When the nasal membrane is rubbed during sutra neti, the sensation vibrates in and through the brain, awakening its entire system, removing all congestions, contractions and depressions. Practise jala neti, followed by sutra neti and ghee neti. Sutra neti has an immediate effect on the memory and concentration centres of the brain.

Ghee neti prevents allergic conditions from occurring around the inflamed mucous membrane. Just as Vicks is inhaled, ghee is inhaled.

Using milk is another type of neti. It is an almost sure cure for various nasal diseases, such as colds, inflammation and sinusitis. It should be done after jala neti and simple pranayama. It has been observed that eye sores, and nasal infections have been successfully cured by milk neti. This is a yogic panacea.

How does neti help general health?

Swami Satyananda: Neti has a subtle influence on the various nerves which end in the nasal passages, such as the olfactory bulb and adjacent nerves which innervate the eyes and ears. Respiration is much easier when the nose is clean and clear, leading to an improved intake of oxygen, improved removal of carbon dioxide and consequently better health.

These effects have a soothing influence on the brain and can help to relieve ailments such as migraine, epilepsy, depression, insomnia, and tension. Neti also helps cure sinusitis, ailments of the eyes, nose and throat, tonsillitis, catarrh, and inflammation of the adenoids and mucous membranes. It leaves a general feeling of lightness and freshness in the head, and removes drowsiness. The benefits of neti kriya are many.

What are the general health benefits of neti?

Swami Niranjanananda: Neti is an ENTE practice – ear, nose, throat, eyes. There are many tiny, sensitive nerves connecting the eyes, ears, mouth, throat and brain. Not only are the sinuses cleared with neti, but at the same time as the water flows, sensations are created in these tiny little nerves and they are stimulated. There are many examples of short-sightedness being rectified with neti, as neti stimulates the optical nerves. Neti can also reduce hearing loss by stimulating the associated nerves. In *Hatharatnavali* (1:40) it says:

> *Kapaalashodhanee chaiva divyadrishtipradaayinee.*
> *Jatroordhvajaatarogadhnaa jaayate netiruttamaa.*
> *Netisvaroopam kathitam shreenivaasena yoginaa.*
>
> This best neti cleanses the frontal sinuses, bestows upon one keen eyesight and destroys the multitude of diseases in the region above the clavicle. Thus, Srinivasa yogi has explained neti.

The sinuses are cleaned, the nose is not blocked, and one can breathe properly. The forehead is stimulated, helping relieve migraine and other types of headaches. Neti cleanses and clears the throat, and the vocal cords and related nadis are activated and influenced.

Neti helps manage headache, eye ache, ear ache, mouth ache, throat ache. Neti is the biggest ENT doctor in the world.

What are the benefits of sutra neti?

Swami Satyananda: Sutra neti gives a frictional massage to the internal mucous membranes of the nose, strengthening the membranes, making them more efficient and more able to effectively condition – that is clean, moisten, disinfect and warm – the air as it enters the nose prior to entering the lungs.

Sutra neti stimulates many of the large number of nerve endings in the nasal passages. This improves the innervation of the various functions of the nose and their connections with the brain.

This stimulation also causes a slight irritation to the mucous membranes, resulting in increased blood circulation in the nose which tends to encourage excessive secretion of mucus for a short period of time. This is beneficial, for it removes any stagnation of blood in the nostrils and flushes out the secretory glands. The organs in the nose are consequently encouraged to function far more effectively. This includes the eyes, since the tear duct outlet in the nose and the blood supplies are closely connected.

Sutra neti is an excellent method of preventing colds or other inflammations of the nose, especially if it is supplemented with jala neti. The nasal passages are rendered more resistant to attack by germs or viruses.

The ideal combination is sutra neti performed in conjunction with jala neti. Jala neti removes the less ingrained obstructions and flushes out the nose, while sutra neti removes the more obstinate foreign bodies and dried up mucus deposits. It is for this reason that it is highly recommend that jala neti be practised immediately after sutra neti to flush out all the particles in the nose and leave it in the cleanest possible condition.

How long does it take to experience the benefits of neti?

Swami Niranjanananda: The benefits of neti are experienced immediately, as it clears the nasal passages and sinuses.

How does sutra neti keep the nostrils healthy?

Swami Niranjanananda: With the practice of sutra neti the mucous membrane is properly massaged, its function is enhanced, blood flow is increased and the blood supply to the nostrils is optimized. The moving thread or catheter exerts pressure on the glandular lining of the nostrils, reducing swelling and inflammation. Any abnormal growth of the nasal bone is reduced due to the friction produced in sutra neti. Thus one gets relief from sinusitis, rhinitis and abnormal growth of the nasal bone by doing this practice.

How does neti help prevent and cure the common cold?

Swami Satyananda: Neti is the best method of preventing and eliminating colds. An effective cure for the common cold has not yet been found. Neti is not foolproof, but it goes a long way to solving the problem. A cold indicates that the body is in a weakened condition. The cold virus flourishes in nerve tissue, particularly the olfactory nerves in the nose. During a cold, neti greatly helps by removing the accumulated mucus in the nose, this being a breeding ground for the cold virus.

Regular practice of neti during good health keeps the nasal passages working at optimum efficiency and thereby helps prevent disease. When one is forced to breathe through the mouth due to a blocked nose, normal filtering of the air does not take place. Breathing through the mouth, or insufficient treatment of the inhaled air due to nasal congestion, encourages the onset of disease by allowing germs to infect the lungs, or by generally weakening the body.

Why is neti more than just cleansing the nose?

Swami Satyananda: Neti is not only cleaning of the nose, it is also irrigating, or cooling, the optic system, the frontal brain and the glottis. By the practice of neti, if it is correctly done with water, rubber catheter, milk, or clarified butter, one can awaken a certain gland which is situated in the interior of the nose behind the mucous membrane.

Why is neti important in swara yoga?

Swami Satyananda: The science of swara yoga maintains that the flow of air in each nostril alternately changes. If one checks the nostrils it will be observed that one is admitting more air than the other. After some time the other nostril will admit the greater amount of air.

In turn, this alternate flow of breath through the two nostrils has a profound influence on a person's energy cycle. It controls one's thinking and physical activity, one's introversion and extroversion: this cycle has a great bearing on mental and physical health.

If one or both of the nostrils is permanently blocked, this natural alternation of breath flow cannot occur, and health suffers. This is another reason why jala neti is so important; it cleans both nostrils and allows the breath to alternate freely between the two.

Why is jala neti helpful for ear ailments?

Swami Satyananda: Many ear ailments are caused by blockage of the eustachian tubes. The ear is divided into three chambers: the outer, middle and inner sections. Sound vibrations are transmitted from the environment through the outer ear and into the middle ear via the eardrum, which also separates the outer ear from the middle ear. There is no direct connection between the two chambers. For perfect hearing the pressure of air in the middle ear must be the same as that outside the body – atmospheric. This is brought about by means of the two eustachian tubes, which connect each ear to the back of the throat. These tubes are about the same diameter as a pencil lead and easily become blocked with mucus deposits. The best way to remove this type of problem is by practising jala neti, as this helps draw blockages out from these tubes.

How does neti benefit the eyes?

Swami Niranjanananda: Jala neti is the best practice for cleansing the eyes and sustaining vision. Jala neti influences the organs and muscles connected with vision. Blood flow in the capillaries supplying the eyes is increased and as a result the eyes receive more blood. This helps remove metabolic waste, such as carbon dioxide, from the eye area. It has been found that disorders of the eyes are often rectified solely with this practice, particularly if the defects are in their initial stages. Additionally, different people have individual experiences. Some may find their headaches go away; others will note their speech develops clarity.

What are the effects of neti on allergies?

Swami Niranjanananda: The effects of neti on allergy are remarkable. There are many types of allergy. Medical science has acknowledged multiple triggers of allergy: smoke, dust, certain fibres, pollen, animal hair and more. One of the causes of respiratory disease, including asthma, is allergy. With the practice of neti these diseases can be cured without any other remedy. Insomnia and tiredness can also be resolved with this practice. It allows the lungs to receive air that has been efficiently cleansed by the nostrils, helping the whole body remain healthy.

How does neti work?

Swami Niranjanananda: Neti is for the head region. The benefits of neti are for problems related to the nose, eyes and ears. The nose is connected to many different nerve endings. The optic nerves are connected with the visual area of the brain, the auditory nerves are connected with the hearing part of the brain, and the olfactory nerves with the sense of smell. All these nerves are located in and around the nostrils and the upper throat.

In the practice of neti, as the water goes through the mucous membrane, it touches all these nerve endings on its way and stimulates them, directly or indirectly. The temperature, force and flow of water stimulate them, causing many people in the initial stages of practising neti to feel tears come to their eyes. Neti removes the impurities, the dust and dirt that are absorbed by the membrane, the excess dryness or wetness, and provides a proper healthy structure to the membrane.

What influence does neti have on the nadis and chakras?

Swami Satyananda: Spiritually, neti aids in the awakening of *ajna chakra*, the third eye. Neti and other kriyas in hatha yoga are intended for the union of ida and pingala nadis.

Does neti prepare the practioner for khechari mudra?

Swami Satyananda: Neti is an important practice, particularly for those who want to practise khechari mudra. In the practice of khechari mudra the tongue is folded back and inserted into the epiglottis.

Does neti kriya have spiritual benefits?

Swami Niranjanananda: With regard to the spiritual benefits of neti kriya, it is said that the practice awakens ajna chakra. With the awakening of ajna chakra the mind becomes calm, there is the experience of one-pointedness and the attainment of concentration. Such a person has a proper understanding of their own actions, and gains subtle insights. In *Gheranda Samhita* (1:50–51) it is written:

> *Vitastimaanam sookshmasootram naasaanaale praveshayet;*
> *Mukhaannirgamayetpashchaat prochyate netikarmakam.*
>
> *Saadhanaannetikaaryasya khechareesiddhimaapnuyaat;*
> *Kaphadoshaa vinashyanti divyadrishtih prajaayate.*
>
> Take a thread half as long as the arm, insert it in the nose and take it out through the mouth. This is called neti karma. (50)
>
> The practice of neti enables one to attain perfection in khechari, elimination of kapha and attainment of divine vision. (51)

In verse 51, Sage Gheranda describes three benefits of neti kriya: the rectification of kapha disorders, the attainment of divine vision, and the attainment of perfection in khechari mudra. Here, "perfection of khechari mudra" is a state of attainment. After perfecting khechari mudra, a yogi achieves complete control over the body and can perceive defects of the body. It helps in attaining the siddhi of astral travelling. Many other siddhis are attained as well.

The term *divya drishti* means 'divine vision' and has been wrongly interpreted as clairvoyance. Clairvoyance is a state of mental achievement whereas divine vision is an experience of an awakened personality. The practice of neti helps in attaining the awakening of the inner personality with the regulation of the ida, pingala and sushumna flows, ultimately resulting in the awakening of the chakras and of kundalini.

How does neti help one attain higher yogic states?

Swami Niranjanananda: Neti provides a state of mental clarity which is useful for the higher practices of yoga. It is not simply the act of pouring water through one nostril and making it come out through the other. It is not only a practice of putting a catheter through one nostril and bringing it out through the mouth. Rather, the physical practice of neti gives birth to an internal state of neti which is the flow of prana shakti in the three channels of ida, pingala and sushumna.

Once the flow in ida and pingala is balanced, the harmony of the two flows will accentuate the flow of sushumna. The awakening of sushumna will, in turn, be responsible for the development of higher mental faculties, leading one's nature towards genius, intuition and creativity.

4

Introduction to Dhauti

WHAT IS DHAUTI?

What is dhauti?

Swami Satyananda: Dhauti is the second kriya of hatha yoga. The word *dhauti* means 'to wash'. Techniques of dhauti are used to clean the alimentary canal, the inner walls of the stomach, intestines and bowel. There are also dhautis for cleaning the ears, eyes and teeth. There are various ways of performing dhauti. When water is used, it is called *jala dhauti*. Sometimes cloth, air, or foodstuffs are also used for the cleaning. Dhauti must be practised under the guidance of a guru.

What are the categories of dhauti?

Swami Niranjanananda: There are four categories of dhauti: *antar* (internal) dhauti, *danta* (head) dhauti, *hrid* (cardiac) dhauti and *moola* (anal) shodhana. Air, water and cloth are the three means of cleansing. Through these practices yogis keep their bodies clean and healthy. In *Gheranda Samhita* (1:13) it is written:

Antardhautirdantadhautirhriddhautirmoolashodhanam
Dhautim chaturvidhaam kritvaa ghatam kurvanti nirmalam.

Antar dhauti, danta dhauti, hrid dhauti and moola shodhana are the four types of dhauti which keep the body clean and healthy.

Antar dhauti means internal cleansing. These practices cleanse the stomach and digestive tract. The literal meaning of *danta dhauti* is cleaning the teeth, but here it means cleansing the frontal region of the head, rather than the literal meaning. The third dhauti is *hrid dhauti*, cleansing of the heart region, which includes the oesophagus and lungs. The fourth is *moola shodhana*, cleansing the base or root portion of the body including the anus, rectum, large intestine and urinary tract.

What types of dhauti are for the digestive system?

Swami Satyananda: There are six major dhautis for cleansing the alimentary canal: *vaman dhauti*, also known as *kunjal*, is washing the stomach by means of vomiting; *vyaghra dhauti* is the technique for a loaded stomach; *varisara dhauti*, popularly known as *shankhaprakshalana*, is a method of cleaning the entire alimentary canal from mouth to anus; *vatsara*, or *vayu dhauti* is a process of cleaning the stomach by air; *agnisara dhauti* is a technique to stimulate the spiritual heat of the body by stimulating the digestive fire and the serpent fire. *Agni* means fire.

PURPOSE

Why is dhauti such an important practice?

Swami Satyananda: The combination of all the practices of dhauti cleans the entire digestive tract and the respiratory tract. Dhauti removes excess and old bile, mucus and toxins, and restores the natural balance of the body's chemical composition, alleviating ailments caused by such imbalances. The various practices help remove infectious bacteria from the mouth, nose, eyes, ears, throat, stomach, intestines and anus.

The results are a reduction of excess fatty tissue and relief from flatulence, constipation, poor digestion and loss of appetite. Dhauti is even said to cure leprosy. Although this disease is not prevalent in many countries today, the point is that even such insidious diseases can be alleviated through this powerful practice. In *Hatha Yoga Pradipika* (2:25) it states:

> *Kaasashvaasapleehakushtham kapharogaashcha vinshatih.*
> *Dhautikarmaprabhaavena prayaantyeva na samshayah.*
>
> There is no doubt that coughs, asthma, diseases of the spleen, leprosy and twenty kinds of diseases caused by excess mucus are destroyed through the effects of dhauti karma.

The *Gheranda Samhita* states that dhauti can cure abdominal ailments and fever. Of course, it is not advisable to practise dhauti during a fever or acute visceral infection. If practised after recuperation, however, dhauti can prevent recurrence of the problem.

What digestive disorders are helped by practising dhauti?
Swami Niranjanananda: The dhauti techniques help to remove many stomach ailments. Indigestion and other abdominal disorders such as constipation, irritable bowel syndrome and hyperacidity can be cured by practising dhauti.

Why is maintaining a healthy digestive system so important in hatha yoga?
Swami Niranjanananda: Emphasis is laid on the cleanliness of the internal organs in all the shatkarma practices, especially those of dhauti. According to yoga, seventy-five per cent of diseases in the human body are caused by disorders in the digestive system, so in the shatkarma practices of dhauti, emphasis has been laid on correcting the digestive system.

There are other causes of ill health such as environmental pollution and bacterial infection, but most health complaints are compounded by problems in the digestive system. If the abdominal organs become weak, food cannot be digested efficiently and constipation, diarrhoea, or liver upsets often occur. Most of the remaining twenty-five per cent of diseases occur due to mental worries and tensions.

In yoga there are different ideas regarding diet and digestion for yoga practitioners and householders. A practitioner who perfects yoga increases the digestive capacity to such an extent that virtually anything can be digested. For householders, a sattwic, regulated and simple diet is recommended as it is difficult to fully control the lifestyle. The aim of hatha yoga is to make the body so strong that it remains totally unaffected by any type of lifestyle, but for a householder that is not a realistic aim.

What is the result of practising dhauti?

Swami Niranjanananda: What is the result of the four practices of dhauti? In the words of Sage Gheranda, *Ghatam kurvanti nirmalam,* they make the body pure.

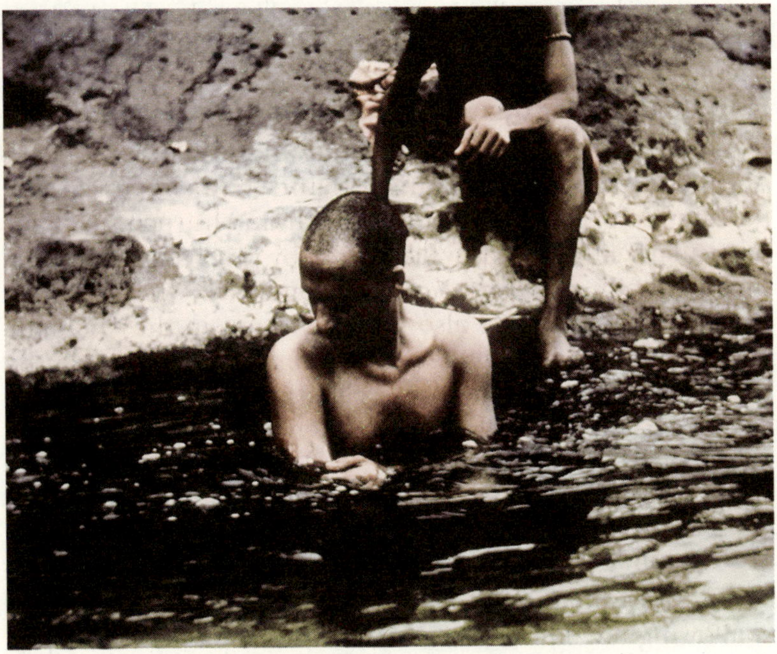

5

Antar Dhauti: Internal Cleansing

GENERAL BENEFITS

What are the benefits of practising antar dhauti?

Swami Sivananda: Those who do any form of antar dhauti have no need of purgatives or laxatives. They never suffer from indigestion or constipation. Those who can fill up their stomach with air can float on water just like a dead body. They can also live on air and water for some days without any food.

How do the antar dhauti practices affect the koshas?

Swami Niranjanananda: The four antar dhauti practices – vatsara, varisara, vahnisara and bahishkrita – are techniques for making the body free from obstructions. They particularly affect the physical body; by practising them, the physical body, *annamaya kosha*, becomes free from disease. Beneficial changes are also brought about in the energetic and mental bodies, *pranamaya* and *manomaya koshas*. By awakening any nerve centre or chakra through shatkarmas, the entire being is profoundly influenced.

VATSARA DHAUTI: CLEANSING WITH AIR

How is antar dhauti practised with air?

Swami Sivananda: Internal cleaning can be done by swallowing air. The stomach is filled with plenty of air. Just as one swallows food little by little, one can swallow air, filling up the stomach and intestines. This is done by hiccough. Then, by contracting the abdominal muscles, the air passes away through the anus as apana vayu. The technique must be learned from a master of this kriya.

What is vatsara dhauti?

Swami Satyananda: *Vatsara dhauti* is a process of cleaning the stomach with air. Vatsara dhauti is performed by breathing in slowly through the mouth in *kaki mudra*, the crow's beak, then swallowing the air into the stomach while expanding the abdomen. This can be done up to ten times or until the stomach is fully expanded, then the air is expelled through the mouth.

Is vatsara dhauti a form of burping?

Swami Satyananda: The subject of burping has long been controversial in various societies throughout the world, although in China and during the middle ages of Europe, it was almost a ritual to end a meal by burping. This showed clearly that one had enjoyed the food. If a person did not burp he was likely to be labeled bad mannered or even a boor. Burping was almost considered an art. This art has been lost in modern societies as it is considered crude and distasteful. Nevertheless, there is a place for the revival of this noble and ancient art.

Under normal circumstances burping brings a wonderful and immediate sense of relief. It is a normal response which no one can avoid; everyone tends to swallow air while eating, as air is trapped in each mouthful of food and accumulates in the stomach. The amount of air swallowed varies greatly with eating habits, but it may be as much as half a litre. A little of this passes into the intestinal tract but most of it is expelled by means of the simple expedient of burping.

Vatsara dhauti uses the same basic process, but instead of introducing air into the stomach by eating food, it is brought in by voluntary effort. In other words, air is sucked into the stomach while inhaling. To many people, especially children, this technique comes almost naturally. In fact, many children already practise it for the fun of hearing the resulting noise on expulsion, without realizing that they are performing an ancient practice of yoga.

The main reason for doing vatsara dhauti is to cleanse the stomach of stale, foul-smelling gases. Also, many processes of digestion improve when there is a liberal supply of oxygen in the stomach. The oxygen seems to encourage the best possible digestion of food; aeration of the stomach aids digestion and eliminates waste gas.

What are the benefits of vatsara dhauti?

Swami Satyananda: It is easy to treat this practice in a rather light-hearted and superficial manner, as it is difficult to be serious and factual about such a maligned subject as burping. However, it must be emphasized that this practice is beneficial. It increases the digestive power of the body by improving the chemical reactions taking place within the stomach. It removes impure and unwanted gases and helps to eliminate and prevent hyperacidity and especially heartburn.

When one considers that a large number of ailments arise from digestive disorders, the necessity for a healthy digestive system becomes obvious. Vatsara dhauti is one method of attaining this end.

What is the purpose of practising vatsara dhauti?

Swami Niranjanananda: Vatsara dhauti cleanses the stomach and intestines by using air. Just as accumulated dust and dirt can be removed by blowing air or using suction, similarly, in the practice of vatsara dhauti air is introduced into the stomach, expelling toxic or foul-smelling gases and wind, and stimulating the digestive system.

In *Gheranda Samhita* (1:16) it says, *dehanirmalakaarakam*, vatsara kriya makes the body clean internally. *Nirmala* means pure, sacred. A pure body results in good health.

Many diseases are associated with digestive problems. Restoring balance to the digestive system benefits overall wellbeing.

Sarvarogakshayakaram dehaanalavivardhakam, this practice destroys all diseases and increases the effectiveness of the digestive fire by enhancing the chemical reactions in the stomach. It expels unwanted gases from the stomach, regulates the production of gastric juices, mucus and acid, and removes irritation and pain caused by acidity in the stomach and oesophagus. If the digestive system is functioning well, digestive juices are produced in the right quantity, excretion of faeces becomes regular and many health problems such as constipation, diarrhoea, peptic ulcers and reflux (heartburn) are reduced.

What are the guidelines for practising vatsara dhauti?

Swami Niranjanananda: Vatsara dhauti can be explained, but it is important to know more than just the technique. For example, which asana should be adopted? One should sit in a meditative asana like padmasana, sukhasana, siddhasana or siddha yoni asana, with the hands placed on the knees and the spine kept straight; it should not be performed while standing. When standing, the intestines are open and air can freely enter them, but when sitting in an asana, the physical position contracts the intestines, causing a type of blockage which keeps the air in the stomach. Therefore, this practice should be done seated in a meditative asana. In *Gheranda Samhita* (1:15) it says:

> *Kaakachanchuvadaasyena pibedvaayum shanaih shanaih*
> *Chaalayedudaram pashchaadvartmanaa rechayechchhanaih.*
>
> Shaping the lips like a crow's beak, slowly, slowly suck in as much air as possible, circulate it inside the abdomen and then gradually expel it completely.

Once seated comfortably, the lips are pursed in the shape of a crow's beak. Air is then swallowed in the same way as drinking water. In pranayama, air is taken into the lungs, but in this practice air is not allowed into the lungs, it is taken straight into the stomach, as if it were water. When water is swallowed, the windpipe automatically closes so that water cannot enter. Gargling also closes off the windpipe, preventing water from entering it. How to close the windpipe at will needs to be learned first; for this, there needs to be control over the muscles of the throat which control closure of the windpipe.

Secondly, how to take air into the stomach needs to be understood. When the air is sucked into the stomach, it is kept inside for a minute or two only, not more. Normal respiration continues. No mention is made of breath retention. Respiration goes on while the air is kept inside the stomach. After one or two minutes the air is slowly released by belching. If the stomach is in an unhealthy state, the expelled air will be foul-smelling, but this is rare.

The speed with which the air enters should be regulated, and not too fast. The mouth should not be open too much as the amount of air sucked into the mouth is the quantity of air swallowed. Gradually more air is taken in and then more again. The speed should be similar to the normal speed of respiration, not like gulping water rapidly. Generally, with the air retained in the abdomen, vahnisara (agnisara kriya) or lauliki (nauli kriya) is performed, rotating the air in the abdomen. After rotation, the air is released.

This practice stimulates the digestive system and removes gas and wind. Normally, an experience of lightness is felt after belching. Vatsara dhauti is a simple practice, which may be done knowingly or unknowingly. When eating, air is often swallowed with food and it enters the stomach. Sometimes it is expelled through the rectum, but mostly it comes out through the mouth in the form of belching. Vatsara dhauti is based on this natural practice. However, air is not accidentally swallowed as at the time of eating, but consciously directed into the stomach.

When is the best time to practise vatsara dhauti?

Swami Satyananda: This practice is most useful when performed just before eating a large or heavy meal, as it stimulates the digestive system. It can be practised as many times as one wants, but once or twice just before eating is sufficient. It can, however, be done at any time of the day, but not during or immediately after a big meal.

When should practising vatsara dhauti be avoided?

Swami Niranjanananda: The rules for this practice are similar to those for other practices. Just as asanas are best done on an empty stomach, this rule is also followed in dhauti, but more strictly, as if there is food in the stomach it will be expelled during the practice. It should always be remembered that asanas, pranayamas, shatkarmas and all the physical practices of yoga should be done on an empty stomach.

If the practice is performed incorrectly without practical knowledge and guidance, there is the possibility of causing harm. It needs to be remembered that not everyone is able to do the higher practices of yoga. Some people may be limited by their physical constitution, reduced physical capacity, or simply due to ageing. An eighty-year-old should not be given heavy duty shatkarmas, but advised to do light practices like pawanmuktasana, nadi shodhana pranayama and yoga nidra. Not all yogic practices are suitable for everyone. The physical capacity, condition and aim of the individual must be considered.

Often when people experience pain in the chest, the cause is wind rather than a heart attack. When wind in the digestive system moves upwards, it can cause a feeling of pressure inside the chest and there may be a slight pain in the heart region. Many people become frightened, mistaking the sensation for a heart attack. That misunderstanding can create so much fear that the pain intensifies. In such a situation vatsara is useful. However, vatsara kriya should not be performed by those who have suffered a heart attack in the past two or three years, and must also be avoided by those who have had heart surgery.

Why isn't the practice of vatsara dhauti more widely known?

Swami Niranjanananda: In *Gheranda Samhita* (1:16) it states that:

> *Vaatasaaram param gopyam deha nirmalakaarakam;*
> *Sarva rogakshayakaram dehaanalavivarddhakam.*
>
> Vatsara is a very secret technique for purifying the body. It destroys all diseases and activates the gastric fire, which helps to digest food.

Vaatasaaram param gopyam means, vatsara is a most secret practice. Why is it secret? There are several reasons. If one thinks about it, all yogic practices are treated as secret, for a number of reasons. No one has complete knowledge of the practical aspect of yoga, and the results of yogic practice are extremely subtle. Also, the result of a practice can never be known by merely learning it from a book. For example, people often try to awaken kundalini by reading about it and sometimes doing the practices as well, but when kundalini starts to stir without proper preparation, such unprepared people can go crazy.

VARISARA DHAUTI: CLEANSING WITH WATER (SHANKHAPRAKSHALANA)

What is varisara dhauti?

Swami Satyananda: Varisara dhauti is a method of cleaning the entire alimentary canal from the mouth to the anus with warm saline water. It is popularly known as *shankhaprakshalana*. Five litres or more of water are drunk and evacuated through the anus. It is a process that must be learned under an expert.

Ancient yogis, such as Sage Gheranda, named this technique of stomach and intestinal wash, *varisara*. *Vari* means water in both Sanskrit and Hindi. *Sara* means 'with essence', or 'pertaining to'. In the term shankhaprakshalana, the word *shankha*, meaning 'conch', is used as the shape of the stomach is shaped like the conch. *Shalana* means 'to wash'. *Prakshalana* means 'to wash completely'.

How is varisara dhauti traditionally practised?

Swami Sivananda: There are some people who can drink plenty of water and pass it through the anus immediately.

The practice of drinking water and quickly passing it out of the anus is called *varisara dhauti* and is also known as *sang pachar kriya*. Nauli and uddiyana bandha should be combined for performance of this exercise.

How can the entire intestinal tract be cleansed?

Swami Niranjanananda: The practice of shankhaprakshalana cleans both the small and large intestines. Shankhaprakshalana is the modern method of varisara dhauti, in the sense that it is acceptable to all and can be practised by everyone, providing there is an awareness of the appropriate climatic and dietary restrictions that have to be followed after the practice.

There are two variations of this practice. One is called *laghoo shankhaprakshalana*, the short form, in which six glasses of warm saline water are drunk, two at a time, followed by the performance of five asanas which loosen up the intestines and allow the water to pass through. The second variation is called *poorna shankhaprakshalana*, the full form, in which a total of sixteen or more glasses of water are drunk in combination with the practice of the same specified asanas. The saline water flushes the whole system by creating pressure, and thoroughly cleans out all the accumulated particles from the intestines. This process also removes the entire mucous lining from the intestine, which makes the digestive system highly sensitive and also increases mental sensitivity.

The effects of shankhaprakshalana include stimulation of the nervous system, improvement of the digestive function, elimination of toxins from the entire system and sensitization of the nadis that link the chakras together. The state of physical purification also helps the pranamaya kosha to reorganize and restructure the flow of prana in the body. The increased sensitivity in the mind and energy is due to the effect of the practice on the pranic body. For this reason many people are physically tired after performing shankhaprakshalana, but still have a lot of energy within them. There is no heaviness in the body; the whole body feels light, as if it is floating.

Which practice of dhauti is best for aiding the elimination of waste from the intestines?

Swami Satyananda: For elimination problems, experience has shown that the best form of dhauti is shankhaprakshalana. With about sixteen glasses (or four to five litres) of warm saline water, the whole alimentary canal is cleaned from top to bottom. Within a period of only one and a half hours, one can be rid of all the fermenting, decomposed mucus in the intestines.

On the intestinal walls there is hard mucus which food sticks to. As this mucus decomposes, it should be expelled. Unfortunately, modern thinking says that when mucus passes there is a disease, and medicine is immediately taken to stop the process, instead of allowing this decomposed mucus to be thrown out by nature's method. When shankhaprakshalana is practised, the large and small intestines are washed clean of this decomposed mucus. When this mucus is completely expelled, a state of cleanliness and health is created in the whole system.

What are the benefits of practising shankhaprakshalana?

Swami Satyananda: Shankhaprakshalana is the best exercise of hatha yoga. Those who practise it have an aura that shines brilliantly. It purifies the body, eliminates all toxins from the stomach and cleans the whole alimentary canal. It also dispels worms from the intestines. Constipation is cleared and diabetes can be cured by this practice. The body becomes light and free from tension.

Why is it important to clean the intestines?

Swami Niranjanananda: Most people never clean their intestines. It is well known that if one does not drink enough water, faeces build up in the large intestine, becoming dry and hard and causing constipation. When a bowel action finally occurs, the delicate lining of the intestine, bowel or anus may be scratched by the hard stool, which can be painful and even cause bleeding.

Even drinking several litres of water daily does not fully clean the stomach and intestines. The water is absorbed through the intestinal walls and flows through the bloodstream to the kidneys where it is excreted as urine. As the water does not pass through the intestines, decaying matter remains trapped in the crevices of the intestines and can cause disease. Shankhaprakshalana overcomes this problem and is a simple cure for constipation. In *Gheranda Samhita* (1:17–18) it is written:

> *Aakantham poorayedvaari vaktrena cha pibechchhanaih*
> *Chaalayedudarenaiva chodaraadrechayedadhah.*
>
> *Vaarisaaram param gopyam dehanirmalakaarakam;*
> *Saadhayettatprayatnena devadeham prapadyate.*
>
> Drink water slowly through the mouth up to the throat. The abdomen is then moved and the water evacuated through the anus. (17)
>
> The technique of varisara dhauti is most secret. It purifies the body. A yogi who perfects this technique attains a divine body. (18)

Shankhaprakshalana makes the body clean and pure. It is the best practice for purification of wastes and disorders of the digestive system. Sage Gheranda says that a yogi who perfects this technique attains *devadeham* – a divine, lustrous, brilliant and light body like that of a god. Through this practice the body can be kept free from all types of diseases.

What are the effects of excess mucus in the intestines?

Swami Satyananda: When the intestines are loaded with decomposed mucus, intestinal peristalsis slows down. When this occurs, decomposition and fermentation of foodstuffs takes place inside the intestines. This means that during the process of assimilation, the body absorbs toxins and the whole body becomes toxic.

Are there a variety of ways to practise shankhaprakshalana?

Swami Satyananda: Almost all ancient texts refer to shankhaprakshalana. In the tradition of hatha yoga and also in ayurveda, different methods of shankhaprakshalana are prescribed for rejuvenation of the body. A few of the varieties are as follows:

1. Pure cold water
2. Water and salt
3. Water and asafoetida
4. Water and garlic essence
5. Water and onion essence
6. Water and bhang (ganja preparation)
7. Water and almond essence
8. Water and lime.

Aside from the above-mentioned variations, there is a mixture of different herbs, numbering seventy-one in all, which may be used for shankhaprakshalana, but only in the presence of an expert teacher. These techniques should never be learned from books only; they must always be done in the presence of an adept. For general purposes, salt water is ideal and should be used.

Can liquids other than salt water be used in shankhaprakshalana?

Swami Satyananda: It is unfortunate that some yogic aspirants have lost sight of the essential and simple practice of shankhaprakshalana and are experimenting with many new variations on the original theme, sometimes with unpleasant results. Some groups of people are substituting lemon water, fruit juice, vegetable soup, and various herbs for salty water. Salt has gained a bad reputation by being associated with high blood pressure and people are afraid to overuse it. The taste of salty water is also deemed undesirable.

The purpose of shankhaprakshalana is to break the old mucous linings. When salt water is introduced into the body there is a certain chemical reaction with the hydrochloric acid and other enzymes. It has been found, even by medical scientists, that salt water is the mildest and safest solution. Salt water cleans the old mucus completely. As a result, the intestines are exposed. One hour later some fat, in the form of ghee, is taken with the first meal to create a temporary lining on the exposed intestines. Salt makes this lining possible. Lemon will not allow it. If there is lemon, fat cannot survive. If one wants to clean a cup which has a lot of fat, soap may fail, but lemon will not fail. Any fruit juice is acidic. It has also been found that salt has a soothing effect on any inflamed areas of the linings of the intestines. Within twenty-four hours of totally cleaning the intestines, new mucus must form on the exposed intestines, otherwise ulcers may develop. Salt is so mild that it does not interfere with the fat that has to stay for the next twenty-four hours. These points must be kept in mind and no mistakes made.

Also, when one is purging twenty to twenty-five times, there is the possibility of dehydration. It doesn't happen to everybody, but it can happen. Can lemon stop dehydration? Is there any scientific theory behind it? People confuse things. In naturopathy they give lemon as it reacts with hydrochloric acid and produces alkalinity, but that is not the purpose of shankhaprakshalana.

If one thinks carefully about what is happening in shankhaprakshalana it becomes clear that anything other than mildly saline water taken in such large quantities is an intense dose. It is easy to overdo things and cause injury. It must be remembered that for each round of the practice two glasses of warm, mildly salty water have to be drunk and five asanas performed eight times each. That is forty movements. This is repeated at least eight to ten times. This is a potent practice and it must be performed carefully and correctly, so as not to further upset the balance of one's system.

The amount of salt assimilated in shankhaprakshalana is quite small. Very little is absorbed as most is excreted through the rectum. This means the salt should not cause any problems in terms of high blood pressure. People with hypertension, however, should not practise shankhaprakshalana.

What is the general procedure for practising shankhaprakshalana?

Swami Satyananda: For this practice five litres of saline water must be prepared. The water must be slightly warmer than body temperature; if it is the same or slightly lower than body temperature, nausea may result. It is necessary to drink two glasses of water at a time, followed by five asanas which are done eight times each, one after the other. The asanas are *tadasana*, palm tree pose, *tiryak tadasana*, swaying palm tree pose, *kati chakrasana*, waist rotation pose, *tiryak bhujangasana*, twisting cobra pose, and *udarakarshanasana*, abdominal stretch pose. This process is repeated until sixteen glasses have been drunk.

As more water is drunk, the process of evacuation becomes very free. In the beginning formed stool will be passed, then liquid stool, then coloured water, and finally clear water. People suffering from chronic constipation may have difficulty evacuating. If so, *padahastasana*, hand-to-foot pose, and *ardha chakrasana*, half-wheel pose, can be added.

After this vigorous cleansing, one rests for ten minutes and then practises kunjal kriya and neti. After that, there must be complete rest, without sleeping, for forty-five minutes, then a preparation of thin khichari made with fine rice, mung dhal and an ounce of ghee is eaten. Khichari should also be taken in the evening, even if one is suffering from diabetes.

After shankhaprakshalana, khichari should be taken within an hour. If kunjal kriya is not successful and the stomach is not emptied, khichari should be taken after fifteen minutes, when the water in the stomach is passed out through evacuation. Water should not be taken until four hours after the completion of the practice. Any amount of khichari can be taken, but it should be taken at the right time without delay, as fat and carbohydrates are necessary to neutralize the effect of acid secretions on the intestinal wall which has been stripped of its mucous lining. Ghee lines the intestinal wall like a layer of grease.

After eating khichari, one should lie down for about two hours rest without sleeping. On the day of the practice, avoid fluctuating temperatures, direct sun or draught. Do not use a fan or take a bath. The day following the practice should also be one of rest. For a weak or diseased person, the rest period should be extended.

What yogic practices need to be known in order to perform shankhaprakshalana?

Swami Niranjanananda: The five asanas, kunjal and neti are part of shankhaprakshalana. After the stomach wash, kunjal and neti are performed. It is only after performing these that the technique of shankhaprakshalana can be said to be complete.

What is the role of the five asanas used in shankhaprakshalana?

Swami Niranjanananda: Five asanas are used in shankhaprakshalana to activate intestinal peristalsis and enhance the cleansing process. When performed in the correct sequence, they work together to systematically open the various intestinal valves between the stomach and the bowels, progressively opening the pyloric valve (at the outlet of the stomach), the ileocecal valve (at the exit of the small intestine) and finally the sphincter which forms the anus, thus encouraging the salt water to flow from the beginning of the intestines to the rectum.

1. *Tadasana*, palm tree pose: The full body stretch in tadasana acts mainly on the stomach and stretches the colon. The oesophagus is held straight, and the stomach and abdomen are alternately compressed and expanded as the body is stretched and released. During inhalation the diaphragm moves downwards, exerting pressure on the abdominal organs. During exhalation, the diaphragm relaxes and the pressure on the abdominal wall relaxes. The muscular orifice, or pyloric valve, between the stomach and the duodenum opens, allowing water to pass through and into the small intestine.

2. *Tiryak tadasana*, swaying palm tree pose: In tiryak tadasana the body is bent sideways. Tiryak tadasana acts on the small intestine and colon. There is expansion on one side of the body and compression on the other. Pressure is exerted first on the intestines on the right side of the abdomen and then on those on the left side. Note that the small intestine starts on the right side of the abdomen. The folded intestines are massaged and water is pushed through them, flushing out any decaying particles.

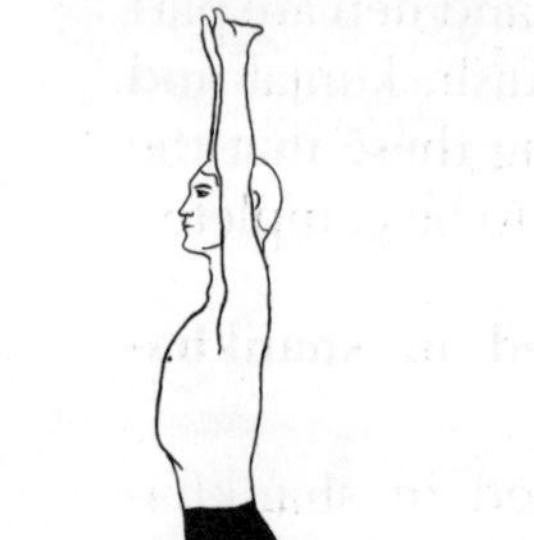

Tadasana

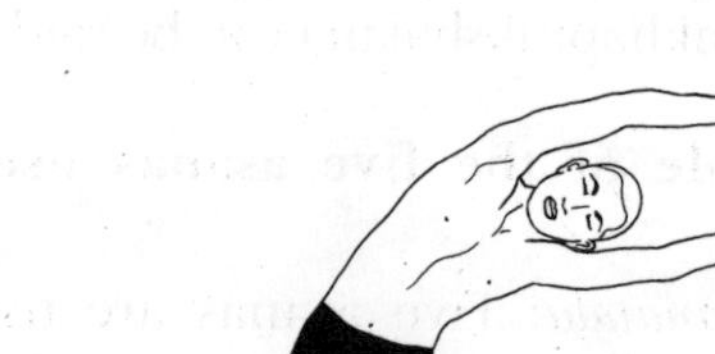

Tiriyak tadasana

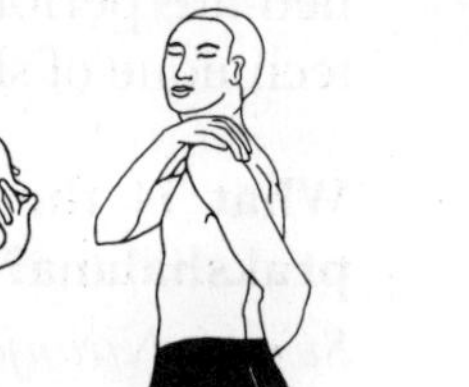

Kati chakrasana

3. *Kati chakrasana*, waist rotating pose: The twisting action of this asana massages the abdominal organs and small intestine, so that the water is pushed through the intestines. The posture should be performed smoothly without undue physical strain.

4. *Tiryak bhujangasana*, twisting cobra pose: This asana is a variation of bhujangasana. It squeezes and massages the stomach and intestines, enabling the ileocecal valve, the shutter between the small and large intestines, to open so that water can enter the large intestine.

5. *Udarakarshanasana*, abdominal stretch pose: *Udara* means abdomen and *akarshana* means pulling or massaging. Udarakarshanasana squeezes and massages the caecum, sigmoid colon and rectum, and also stimulates the urge to defecate. The lower abdomen and digestive organs are alternately stretched and compressed, encouraging water to move through the large intestine, thereby expelling waste. Note that the twist is first to the right to compress the ascending colon, then to the left to compress the descending colon, following the direction of intestinal peristalsis.

In these practices an effort is made to move the water through the oesophagus, stomach and intestines under pressure, and then expel it. The gastrointestinal tract is shaped like a conch, *shankha*. Just as a conch is cleaned by rotating water inside it, this practice has been named

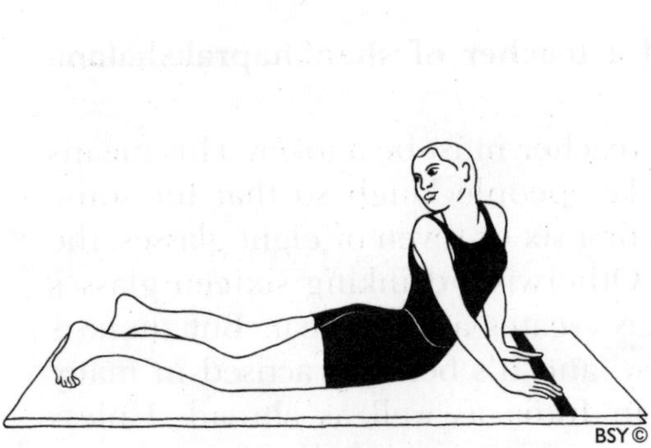

Tiriyak bhujangasana

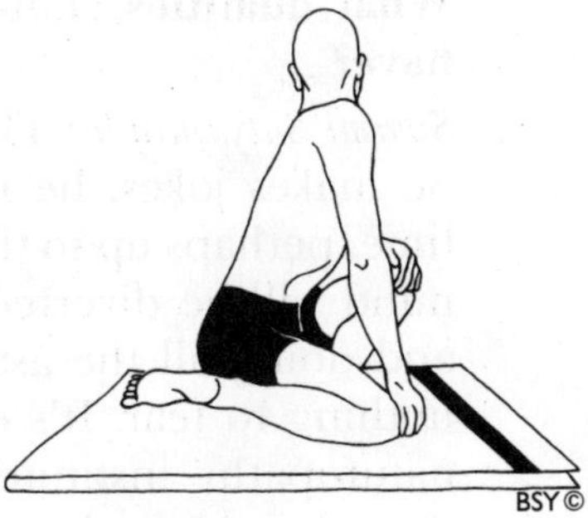

Udarakarshanasana

shankhaprakshalana as the stomach and intestines are cleansed by filling them with water, moving the water through and then expelling it.

What needs to be known about the digestive system when practising shankhaprakshalana?

Swami Niranjanananda: It is important to understand the structure of the digestive system. The digestive tract consists of a long tube from the mouth to the anus called the alimentary canal, which includes the oesophagus, stomach and small and large intestines. The walls of the digestive tract are made of specialized muscles arranged in layers. When the intestinal muscles contract, a rippling movement results and peristalsis occurs. The contents of the digestive system are pushed forward through the digestive tract towards the anus. This rippling contraction resembles the movement of an earthworm.

The intestines are more than six metres long, and are coiled to fit into the abdominal cavity. The inner walls of the digestive system are lined with specialized tissue to allow digestion and absorption to occur. In order to increase the surface area available for absorption, the lining of the small intestine contains circular folds of tissue and the wall of the large intestine is puckered with bulges. However, this also means that particles of semi-digested food or faeces can lodge within the intricate folds of the intestinal lining and decay.

What qualities should a teacher of shankhaprakshalana have?

Swami Satyananda: The teacher must be a joker. This means he makes jokes, he makes people laugh so that for some time, perhaps up to the first six or seven or eight glasses, the mind will be diverted. Otherwise, drinking sixteen glasses and doing all the asanas creates a lot of fear. But there is nothing to fear. It's easy, and it's being practised in many naturopathy institutes in India as well as abroad. Unless there is a medical reason, everyone can do it.

Why are there so many rules for shankhaprakshalana?

Swami Satyananda: The practice of shankhaprakshalana involves the use of water, salt, asana, khichari and ghee. The rules and regulations laid down for the practice are simple and straightforward. They are designed to give maximum results with minimum fuss and problems so that the sadhaka can get on with higher work.

How important is preparation for shankhaprakshalana?

Swami Satyananda: Shankhaprakshalana, if it is properly done, is the easiest of practices. Nevertheless, preparation is important. Before doing shankhaprakshalana the yoga postures should be practised for some time, and also kunjal and neti kriyas.

What are the general guidelines for practising shankhaprakshalana?

Swami Satyananda: Never practise shankhaprakshalana alone. Never allow the body to be exposed to contrasting weather or temperatures below that of the body on the day of practising shankhaprakshalana. It is essential that one has a complete day of rest when doing shankhaprakshalana. If one is ill or in a weakened condition, extend the time of rest.

When should shankhaprakshalana be practised?

Swami Satyananda: Cleansing of the body through shankhaprakshalana should take place according to the seasons prevailing in the country. When the season changes from hot to cold, there is a corresponding change in the whole body. The heating and cooling system, like a thermostat, shifts as the seasons change. At this time shankhaprakshalana should be practised. It should be practised in warm weather; chill must be avoided. The temperature of the atmosphere should be a little above that of the body. It can be performed twice a year at the change of seasons.

Shankhaprakshalana should be practised in the early morning on an empty stomach.

How often can shankhaprakshalana be practised?

Swami Niranjanananda: The weather plays a significant role in the practice of shankhaprakshalana. It must not be performed during extremely cold or extremely hot weather, nor during cloudy, windy or rainy weather. The best time to practise is at the change of the seasons.

Shankhaprakshalana can be performed at intervals of six months, i.e. once or twice a year, when there is a change of seasons; for example, when winter is changing into summer. *Kapha*, mucus, accumulates in the body during winter and starts dissolving and being evacuated when winter is over. This practice can be undertaken when coughing or kapha develops in the chest after winter. According to the seasons in India, it is best to perform shankhaprakshalana in spring (March) and in September, after the rainy season, when temperatures are moderate prior to the onset of colder weather.

In each country one must consider the most suitable time to perform this practice. It should not be performed more than twice a year.

Should one's regular asana practice be performed before shankhaprakshalana?

Swami Niranjanananda: Remember that the physical body has a limit, and for the optimum results it should not be tired during purification practices. Therefore, one's regular asana practice should not be performed on the morning of practising shankhaprakshalana. The practice itself includes many different movements and the internal organs are stimulated into activity, passing water ten, twenty, thirty times. Just constantly running to the toilet is taxing on the body. The more relaxed one is, the easier it will be for the body to respond, but if the body is already tired from performing asanas previously, the system will be cleaned, but it will take longer for the body to recuperate. So – no asana prior to the practice itself.

How is the water be prepared for shankhaprakshalana?

Swami Niranjanananda: The water drunk during this practice should be lukewarm, not hot or cold. Cold water causes constriction of the blood vessels that supply the digestive tract. Hot water is also contra-indicated as it would burn the lining of the gut.

There is an important reason for adding salt. The body cannot absorb salt water easily. When plain water is drunk, it is absorbed through the intestines into the body, and any excess is eliminated in urine. If salty water is drunk, much of it is not absorbed and therefore it comes out via the anus.

It should be remembered that during shankhaprakshalana, water should not be drunk in excess or one may feel like vomiting.

How long does it take to practise shankhaprakshalana?

Swami Niranjanananda: Even though the actual practice is completed in two to three hours, to complete varisara dhauti it takes two days. One should rest for the whole day and the next day. If this is not possible, the practice should not be undertaken. Note there are extensive dietary restrictions for a week and it takes an entire month to gradually return to a full vegetarian diet.

Can shankhaprakshalana be performed at home?

Swami Satyananda: It is recommended that the full course of shankhaprakshalana be performed in an ashram setting where expert guidance is given and strict controls can be exercised over the saline water, the practice itself and the diet following it. If attempting the practice outside of an ashram, do it under guidance and remember, follow the guidelines written in the texts carefully. The ancient yogis, following the instructions of their gurus, knew from experience what they were talking about.

How much rest is needed after practising shankhaprakshalana?

Swami Niranjanananda: On completing the practices, it is essential to rest completely in shavasana for forty-five minutes. This allows the digestive system to revitalize itself following the expulsion of impurities. During this time one should not drink water, bathe, or walk around. Sleep must be avoided as a headache or cold may result. Sometimes people think they are developing a fever as the body temperature can rise after drinking the lukewarm water and sweating may occur, but shankhaprakshalana does not cause fever. Nevertheless, it is important to keep the body warm and comfortable during the rest period.

After eating the first meal, further rest is essential, but it is important not to sleep for at least three hours after this initial meal in order to obtain the full benefits of the practice. Sleeping during this period can lead to lethargy and headache. Complete rest is needed for the remainder of the day. On the following day one should continue to rest and eat khichari. Both physical and mental work should be avoided. If such rest is not possible, the practice should not be done.

Why is fasting advised against following shankhaprakshalana?

Swami Satyananda: Some people believe that fasting after shankhaprakshalana will aid elimination. They are missing the whole point of rebalancing the energies and will debilitate the whole manipura chakra system by straining it in this way.

What are the dietary rules immediately after practising shankhaprakshalana?

Swami Niranjanananda: After resting in shavasana for forty-five minutes, a specially prepared meal of khichari must be eaten. It is important to have light meals after shankhaprakshalana so that there is no extra load on the digestive system. Khichari is light and easy to digest. It is made with good quality, short grain white rice and mung dhal to which *ghee*, clarified butter, is liberally added. These three components help to restore correct digestive function. The ghee should be warmed and melted, so that particles are not floating on the surface. A little *haldi*, turmeric, can also be added to khichari, but no salt. The final preparation is semi-liquid.

The specially prepared khichari is eaten immediately on completion of the forty-five minute rest period, and again for the late afternoon or evening meal, about six hours after the first special meal. The stomach must be filled to capacity at both meals even if there is no feeling of hunger. This relines the intestines and provides bulk, assisting the intestines to resume peristalsis. The stomach is completely empty after the practice and by eating a large quantity of khichari with ghee, the lining of the gut, which was removed by the salty lukewarm water, is replaced with a fatty film. The rice creates mucus, which also protects the inner lining of the alimentary canal. The lentils provide an easily digestible source of protein. Water should not be drunk, but if it is essential, only have one or two sips of warm water.

What dietary rules should be followed in the days after shankhaprakshalana?

Swami Niranjanananda: The following rules must be strictly followed. Those who are unable to follow these food restrictions should not practise shankhaprakshalana.

For seven days one must not eat spicy, acidic, rich or chemically processed foods. Avoid milk and milk products, sweets, tea, coffee, salads and fruits, especially acidic fruits such as lemons. Cigarettes, tobacco, paan, khaini, zarda and other intoxicants such as betel nut are prohibited. Do not take oil, condiments, chilli, pickle, papad or chutney with food.

Take simple, sattwic well-cooked food, such as chapati, khichari, rice and lentils, and bland root vegetables or grains. The lighter the diet, the better. The efficacy of the digestive system needs to be increased gradually by initially taking food which is light, pure and simple. Avoiding foods which are not easily digestible is essential, otherwise the healthy, fresh lining growing in the gut will be destroyed.

Shankhaprakshalana is essential for non-vegetarians. Meat takes longer to digest and so the digestive fire needs to be really effective. Regular meat eating weakens the digestive power and shankhaprakshalana becomes essential to increase the digestive capacity. Eating meat of any kind is prohibited for forty days after the practice.

After shankhaprakshalana the stomach is vulnerable and sensitive like that of a new born baby and extra care should be taken to protect it. Strong allopathic medicines should be avoided for forty days. Alcohol and tobacco products are also prohibited. Not following these rules is as good as playing with one's life.

The aim of shankhaprakshalana is to expel waste from the body and clean the whole digestive tract. These dietary restrictions ensure that the maximum benefits are gained from the practice.

When do bowel movements become normal after practising shankhaprakshalana?

Swami Niranjanananda: Quite often practitioners do not pass stools for two to three days after shankhaprakshalana. This is not constipation. It means that the digestive tract was completely empty and it is taking a long time for the khicheri or other food to travel through the six metre long intestines. Therefore, whether stools are passed or not, do not worry.

Why do some people have unusual experiences after shankhaprakshalana?

Swami Niranjanananda: Many people tend to have unusual experiences after the practice of shankhaprakshalana, as the whole body becomes internally clean like that of a newborn baby; it is totally clean and purified with all the toxins eliminated. All the junk is out, whether from the stomach, upper tract or intestines. This state of physical purification leads to a feeling of floating, lightness, vitality, strength, and dynamism; this experience lasts for many days. When that type of purification is achieved, all physical disturbances, imbalances and distractions automatically stop, and the body becomes receptive to the process of meditation.

In this state the body responds to the experience of meditation as there is no internal imbalance and such a state of purity brings about deep concentration. A lot of mental conflicts and problems simply disappear after practising hatha yoga.

What is laghoo shankhaprakshalana?

Swami Satyananda: The Sanskrit word *laghoo* means 'short', 'condensed' or 'concise'. The word *shankha* means 'conch' or 'shell' and *prakshalana* means 'to wash' or 'to clean thoroughly'. The word shankha is intended to represent and describe the intestine, with its cavernous and coiled shape. Therefore, the term *laghoo shankhaprakshalana* means, the short intestinal wash.

Do laghoo and poorna shankhaprakshalana have different purposes?

Swami Satyananda: The two practices have slightly different purposes: poorna shankhaprakshalana is intended to completely empty and clean the whole digestive system, whereas laghoo shankhaprakshalana is only intended to encourage normal functioning of the intestines.

What are the benefits of laghoo shankhaprakshalana?

Swami Satyananda: People with digestive problems such as constipation, flatulence, acidity, indigestion and other digestive maladies are advised to practise this technique. Laghoo shankhaprakshalana is an excellent method of purifying the body, and of preventing or helping to remove a diverse number of ailments.

Expert guidance should be sought to find out whether it will help to remove particular ailments.

How does laghoo shankhaprakshalana compare with the action of laxatives?

Swami Satyananda: In laghoo shankhaprakshalana, the salt water acts as a lubricant and loosens the stool. Here is an analogy; when there is ingrained crust, stains or coating on the inside of a pot, the first treatment is to soak it for some time in hot water. This loosens up the encrustation, eventually allowing it to be removed easily. The salt water acts in a similar way within the intestines, leaving them clean and free from obstruction.

The salt water does not directly stimulate the nerves. Normally, it is movement and bulk of stool that acts as a trigger, stimulating the nerves which activate peristalsis. The salt water encourages the hardened or blocked stool to move, prompting the nerves to carry out their normal functions. No direct nerve stimulation is involved as it is with laxatives. A further point worth noting is that the salt water does not in itself lead to complete evacuation of the bowels, which is one of the major drawbacks associated with laxatives. Those who are currently using some form of laxative, are advised to adopt laghoo shankhaprakshalana in order to reduce this dependency.

When are shankhaprakshalana and laghoo contra-indicated?

Swami Satyananda: The contra-indications are the same for both practices. People with heart or kidney problems, or high blood pressure, should not do these practices. Those suffering from any medical condition should seek guidance from their doctor before attempting either form, especially if taking medication, as the medication may need to be suspended after poorna shankhaprakshalana. If this is not medically advisable, poorna shankhaprakshalana should not be practised. Laghoo can be practised instead. These practices should also be avoided during pregnancy.

What precautions should be observed when practising laghoo?

Swami Satyananda: After completing the practice wait for half an hour before eating. It must be emphasized that one should not, under any circumstances, try to force a bowel movement. This is the easiest way to develop piles. The bowel movement should be natural.

Are there any dietary restrictions before or after practising laghoo?

Swami Satyananda: Laghoo should be practised in the morning when the stomach is completely empty, before any food or drink is taken. There are no special food restrictions and no special food has to be taken following this practice, although a light vegetarian diet is preferable for that day.

On completion of the practice, one must rest for half an hour before taking any food or drink. Greater benefits are derived by combining this practice with a light diet.

How often should laghoo be practised?

Swami Satyananda: Laghoo can be practised once a week for general purposes. In cases of constipation, however, it may be practised daily until the condition improves.

VAHNISARA DHAUTI: AGNISAR KRIYA

What is vahnisara dhauti?

Swami Satyananda: *Vahnisara*, or *agnisara dhauti*, is a kriya which involves moving the 'fire' in the body. *Vahni* and *agni* mean 'fire'. *Sara* means 'essence', and *dhauti* means 'cleansing action'. Of course, there is no fire as such in the stomach, but the essence or nature of fire can be

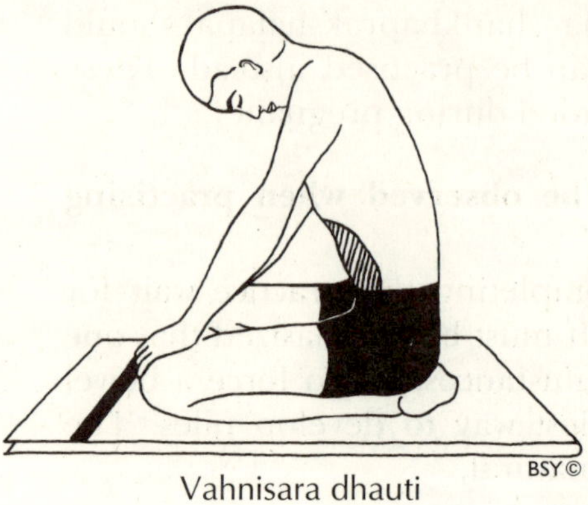

Vahnisara dhauti

compared to the digestive process; the 'essence of fire' is located in the navel region.

If the abdominal organs are not working properly, then the digestive fire only smoulders. When digestion is not as good as it should be, the fire needs to be fanned or stoked. In other words, the process of digestion needs to be kindled and aroused to encourage the best possible digestive power. Agnisar kriya does just this: through continued expansion and contraction of the abdominal muscles, intestinal peristalsis is stimulated, making the digestive fire blaze.

How is agnisar kriya described in the classical texts of hatha yoga?

Swami Satyananda: Agnisar kriya is well known and discussed in the ancient yogic texts. Few details of the practice are given, however, as in the tradition it would be taught by a guru or teacher to his disciple with personal instructions. In *Gheranda Samhita* (1:19–20) agnisar kriya and its benefits are described:

Naabhigranthim meruprishthe shatavaaram cha kaarayet;
Agnisaaramiyam dhautiryoginaam yogasiddhidaa.

Udaraamayajam tvaktvaa jatharaagnim vivarddhayet;
Eshaa dhautih paraa gopyaa devaanaamapi durlabhaa;
Kevalam dhautimaatrena devadeham bhaveddhruvam.

Retaining prana vayu, pull the navel against the spinal column one hundred times. This enables agnisara dhauti to be performed. Diseases of the abdomen are removed and the digestive fire is stimulated. (19)

> This cleansing practice is most secret and is unknown even to the divine beings. By merely doing this practice the body becomes healthy and beautiful, there is no doubt about that. (20)

Of course, it should not be assumed that the text strictly means the navel should be contracted one hundred times; it means that it should be practised as many times as possible without over-exertion. Furthermore, the text should not be taken literally when it says that the practice is unknown to higher beings. This merely implies that the practice is a good one but is rarely practised as few people know of it. The text also indicates that the ancient yogis were fully aware of the benefits of the practice.

How important is vahnisara dhauti in the progression of dhauti practices?

Swami Niranjanananda: Agnisara kriya or vahnisara dhauti is the third practice in the sequence of antar dhauti, and an important one. It cleanses the stomach and internal organs with the help of the fire or heat of *jatharagni*, the digestive fire.

The preceding dhauti practices of vatsara and varisara, use air and water to make the body free from disease. In this practice expansion and contraction of the abdomen take place, massaging all the abdominal organs and enhancing their digestive capacity.

Why should vahnisara dhauti be practised?

Swami Satyananda: Vahnisara, or agnisar dhauti is a simple technique, yet it is highly effective in curing functional and organic disorders of the various systems of the body. Agnisara kriya stimulates the appetite and improves the digestion. It massages the abdomen, strengthens the abdominal muscles and encourages optimum health of the abdominal organs.

Agnisar dhauti is a technique to stimulate the spiritual heat of the body by stimulating the digestive fire and the serpent fire. Agnisara kriya stimulates the five pranas, especially samana, and raises the energy levels markedly. It alleviates depression, dullness and lethargy.

Why is agnisar kriya an important practice for the abdominal organs?

Swami Satyananda: Abdominal malfunctions are common and are often due to lack of exercise and inadequate massage of the internal organs. Many people spend long periods of time sitting motionless doing office work, studying, watching television and doing other activities that require little or no physical effort. This leads to laziness and sluggishness of the entire body, including the abdominal organs. For this reason, the organs become inefficient and unable to perform their basic functions properly, leading to general bad health, whether conspicuous or inconspicuous.

In the case of the abdominal organs, sluggishness leads to indigestion, constipation, kidney and liver problems and various other abdominal ailments. There may be other factors involved, but certainly inefficiency of the organs is a major one. Agnisar kriya is a powerful method to counteract this condition, as it vigorously contracts and expands the abdomen, giving the internal organs the massage and exercise they require in order to function in the best way.

How does agnisara kriya benefit the digestive system?

Swami Niranjanananda: Agnisara kriya promotes the correct secretion of digestive juices and allows optimum assimilation of nutrients from food. Stomach worms can also be destroyed. It prevents and removes disorders of the digestive system such as constipation, indigestion, hyperacidity, hypoacidity, irritable bowel syndrome, pitta imbalance and flatulence. Agnisar kriya balances the abdominal organs.

What posture is used for agnisar kriya?

Swami Satyananda: One can assume various postures to perform agnisar kriya: it can be done from the standing position, from vajrasana or from padmasana. Those who are able to should practise while sitting in vajrasana or padmasana. Otherwise, adopt a standing position, which is equally good.

How many rounds of agnisar kriya should be practised?

Swami Satyananda: Beginners may find this practice difficult and quickly become tired due to lack of voluntary control over the abdominal muscles. The muscles must be slowly and gradually developed over a period of time.

Three rounds of ten abdominal contractions and expansions are sufficient at first. With regular practice, up to fifty abdominal movements may be performed with each round, taking a few moments rest after each round. The time of breath retention should be gradually increased over a period of time. When the muscles become stronger the duration of each round as well as the number of rounds can be increased according to individual capacity. There should be no strain.

How does agnisar kriya prepare one for more advanced practices?

Swami Satyananda: In various yogic practices reasonable control over the abdominal muscles and the ability to manipulate the front wall of the abdomen are required. Most people lack this ability. Agnisar kriya is an excellent preliminary practice to gradually develop effective control of these muscles, while at the same time gaining many other related physical benefits.

Agnisar kriya is useful as a preparation for kapalbhati and bhastrika pranayamas. Sustained practice of agnisara prepares one for *uddiyana bandha*, the abdominal lock. When uddiyana is perfected, one can easily take up nauli. It is a practice in which the entire group of abdominal muscles is toned.

When should agnisar kriya be practised?

Swami Satyananda: Agnisara kriya should be practised early in the morning after going to the toilet and before eating.

The stomach should never be exercised when it is digesting. Practise agnisar kriya after asanas.

During summer months, agnisar kriya should be performed with care as it may raise the body heat and blood pressure excessively. During this period, it should always be followed by a cooling pranayama, such as sheetkari or sheetali.

What precautions should be observed when practising vahnisara dhauti?

Swami Niranjanananda: Agnisara kriya stimulates the nervous system, which places a lot of pressure on the cardiovascular system, abdominal walls and respiratory system. For this reason it should not be performed by anyone suffering from heart disease, high blood pressure, cancer, abdominal ulcers, hernia, asthma or severe respiratory disease. During pregnancy it is contra-indicated, but after delivery it is said to be useful. People with an overactive thyroid gland or chronic diarrhoea should not do this practice.

A healthy body is essential for achieving perfection in the performance of shatkarma practices. The shatkarmas should be undertaken only after ascertaining the capacity of the body. To perfect this practice it is imperative to receive instructions from a guru, otherwise harm may result.

Where should one hold the awareness during the practice of agnisar kriya?

Swami Satyananda: Awareness at the physical level should be on synchronizing the breath rhythmically with the abdominal movement. For spiritual purposes, awareness should be on manipura chakra.

How does agnisara kriya influence the pranic system?

Swami Niranjanananda: Agnisara kriya or vahnisara dhauti is an important practice in relation to prana and kundalini yoga, as it awakens manipura chakra. Mooladhara and swadhisthana are the two chakras in which kundalini shakti can be awakened, but may again fall asleep. Once kundalini shakti reaches manipura, however, it never again becomes inactive. This is the belief according to kundalini yoga. It is also said that the pranas are only awakened in the body after awakening manipura chakra.

Externally no changes may be noticed in a practitioner's life when efforts are made to awaken mooladhara and swadhisthana chakras, but some difficult mental and emotional situations have to be faced, such as excitement, worry, attachment, and sorrow. Here the scriptural principles of yoga are being discussed, not the scientific explanation for the awakening of kundalini. Anatomically, when agnisara kriya is practised, the nerves and glands of the navel region are stimulated. This activation in the solar plexus at manipura chakra directly affects the brain, and pranic activity is experienced in the body. Laxity, laziness and distress are no more.

How does agnisar kriya affect one's energy levels?

Swami Satyananda: Agnisar kriya stimulates the five pranas, especially samana, and raises the energy levels markedly. It alleviates depression, dullness and lethargy.

Can agnisar kriya help people become more extroverted?

Swami Niranjanananda: Agnisara kriya is ideal for people with mental disturbances which cause a high degree of introversion, as it activates the nervous system. For example, moderate performance of agnisar kriya can remove depression for three or four hours.

Why is agnisar kriya not commonly known?

Swami Niranjanananda: In *Gheranda Samhita* (1:20) vahnisara dhauti is said to be such a secret practice that even the gods do not know it: "This cleansing practice is most secret and is unknown even to the divine beings."

It might be wondered what is so secret about moving the abdomen backward and forward, but when it is practised, one realizes how much control is needed to do it correctly. A person who does not possess control over the body cannot do this practice. It is also said that by practising this dhauti alone, one attains a divine body.

BAHISHKRITA DHAUTI: RECTAL CLEANING

Who should practise bahishkrita dhauti?

Swami Satyananda: Bahishkrita dhauti is difficult unless one is an extremely advanced hatha yoga practitioner. It involves standing navel-deep in clean water, pushing out the rectum and washing it in the hands. In *Gheranda Samhita* (1:22–24) this dhauti is described:

> *Naabhimagnajale sthitvaa shaktinaadeem visarjayet;*
> *Karaabhyaam kshaalayennadeem yaavanmalavisarjanam.*
>
> *Taavatprakshaalya naadeem cha udare veshayetpunah;*
> *Idam prakshaalanam gopyam devaanaamapi durlabham;*
> *Kevalam dhautimaatrena devadeho bhaved dhruvam.*
>
> *Yaamaardha dhaaranaashakteem yaavanna dhaarayennarah;*
> *Bahishkritam mahaddhautistaavachchaiva na jaayate.*
>
> Standing in water up to the navel, push out the rectum (shakti nadi) and wash it, removing the waste products. When the nadi is clean, draw it in again. (22)
>
> This cleansing practice of dhauti is very secret. It is not even accessible to the gods. Just by practising this dhauti, one attains a body like that of a divine being. (23)
>
> It is not possible to practise bahishkrita mahadhauti until the ability to retain air in the abdomen for up to one and a half hours has been developed. (24)

What is bahishkrita dhauti?

Swami Niranjanananda: The fourth practice of antar dhauti is *bahishkrita dhauti*, which is similar to vatsara dhauti in that air is used. *Bahir* means outside, and *krit* means doing or taking out. In this practice both the large and small intestines are cleansed with the help of air and water.

After gaining proficiency in the first stage of the practice (with air), the second half of the technique involves standing in water up to the navel and sucking water in through the anus by means of ashwini mudra. When water enters, it is retained and then expelled so that any waste product in the bowel and around the anus is removed. Next, a little ghee or oil is taken on a finger and applied around the anus. The entire process takes place in the water. The full technique is known as *mahadhauti*.

Sage Gheranda cautions that mahadhauti should only be undertaken if the breath can be retained in the abdomen for over one and a half hours, otherwise it is dangerous for the body. Mahadhauti, therefore, should not be performed by everyone. Also, during the practice one should be able to breathe comfortably at the rate of one breath per minute. Therefore, pranayama and other preliminary yoga practices must first be perfected.

How is bahishkrita dhauti with air practised?

Swami Niranjanananda: Bahishkrita dhauti is described in *Gheranda Samhita* (1:21):

> *Kaakeemudraam shodhayitvaa poorayedudaram marut;*
> *Dhaarayedardhayaamam tu chaalayedadhovartmanaa;*
> *Eshaa dhautih paraa gopyaa na prakaashyaa kadaachana.*
>
> Purse the lips like the beak of a crow, take in air through the mouth, filling the abdomen. Retain the air for one and a half hours in the abdomen, then circulate it and expel it through the rectum. It is top secret and is called bahishkrita dhauti.

Kaakeemudraam shodhayitvaa poorayedudaram marut, adopt a facial mudra similar to kaki mudra and inhale so that air fills the abdomen. In the practice of kaki mudra the lips are pursed and air is drawn in through the mouth in a similar way to drinking water. The air is then retained in the abdomen.

In vatsara dhauti normal breathing is practised while retaining the air in the abdomen for a short while before releasing it by belching. In bahishkrita dhauti there is a difference which is explained in the second line of the verse, *dhaarayedardhayaamam tu chaalayedadhovartmanaa*, the air is to be retained in the stomach for half a yama.

Dhaarayed-ardha-yaamam means, hold it for half a yama. In yogic literature the twenty-four hours are divided into yamas. One *yama* is equal to three hours. Half a yama is one and a half hours. Many texts have commented that this means breathing is not allowed for one and a half hours, but it is not possible to retain the breath for so long. Rather it means that the air should be kept in the stomach and alimentary canal for that length of time. It is imperative that these verses are understood in the right perspective.

The air retained in the stomach does not escape through the throat due to the sphincter between the oesophagus and the stomach. *Chaalayedadhovartmana* implies the air is to be moved around inside by churning the abdomen and then expelled through the anus.

In order to perfect this practice, it is necessary to master pranayama. The process is explained here in only a few words. Respiration should actually be kept to a bare minimum once the air has been taken in and retained in the stomach; the slower the respiration, the better. Normally, a person breathes in and out eleven to fifteen times per minute. For this practice, however, the practitioner should be able to take just one respiration per minute; inhalation and exhalation should take thirty seconds each.

This control over respiration is not possible without perfecting the preliminary practices of pranayama. When pranayama is practised, it takes only a little effort to hold the inhalation and exhalation for this duration. Beyond this duration, breathlessness is experienced and it is necessary to take a deep breath in. Such an imbalance should not occur during bahishkrita dhauti; instead, the body should be in a state of complete relaxation, without any physical, muscular or respiratory excitement.

When air is retained in the abdomen for one and a half hours, it is imperative that the practitioner has full control over the stomach, oesophagus and intestines; otherwise the air will leak out of the body through the anus or in the form of belching.

While the air is retained, it is important to perform four of the asanas used in shankhaprakshalana: practising tadasana, tiryak tadasana, kati chakrasana and tiryak bhujangasana pushes the air down the intestines just as water is pushed down in shankhaprakshalana. After performing the asanas, one must go to the toilet as the air pressure which builds up inside the body is released quickly and waste products need to be expelled. In this way, through the medium of air, the intestines are cleaned and diseases of the digestive tract can be removed.

However, a normal person cannot practise bahishkrita dhauti. In reality, it is true to call it a secret practice. *Eshaa dhautih paraa gopyaa,* this dhauti is a highly secret practice, *na prakaashyaa kadaachana,* which should never be taught to the general public. This statement is true. Even accomplished hatha yogis may experience great difficulty performing bahishkrita dhauti.

How does bahishkrita dhauti with water influence the nadis and chakras?

Swami Niranjanananda: Bahishkrita dhauti, the last practice of antar dhauti taught in Gheranda Samhita, is extremely difficult to practise. It is also called *mahadhauti,* the great dhauti, or *prakshalana dhauti,* washing the rectum. Before practising this dhauti it is important to understand the subtle anatomy of the body. In general physiology there is knowledge of the nerves, whereas yogic physiology deals with the more subtle nadis or flows of energy in the body.

Bahishkrita dhauti is a difficult practice, but as it is described in yoga texts it is essential to discuss it. It needs to be clear that even if a practice is difficult, it always has an aim. In this case, part of that aim is to influence particular nadis and chakras.

According to yogic physiology, there are 72,000 nadis in the body, through which a subtle force or *prana shakti* flows. These nadis not only control the flow of blood and the carriage of sensations between the body and brain, but also the flow of power or energy in the body.

The chief nadis originate from mooladhara chakra. In yoga there are special practices for the anus, and the sexual and urinary apparatus. For example, mudras and bandhas awaken nerve fibres, creating sensations and introducing vibrations in different areas of the body where energy knots and nerve plexuses exist. Of the many nerves and nadis originating from and terminating in the mooladhara region, some extend up towards the spine, and some descend from the spine.

Vajra nadi starts on the left side of the anus and is directly related to the sexual and digestive systems, and also to the sciatic nerve. In sciatica, pain starts in the lower back and radiates down one or both legs. Sciatic pain indicates that there is an obstruction or blockage somewhere in vajra nadi, and that the sensations are not flowing as they should.

Shakti nadi is sometimes translated as meaning the rectum and *bahishkrita dhauti* is primarily a practice for cleansing shakti nadi. According to yogic science, shakti nadi starts from the right side of the anus and goes up to mooladhara and swadhisthana chakras, joining pingala nadi at swadhisthana chakra. Pingala nadi carries the solar force or prana shakti. When the finger is inserted and ghee applied, a little water also enters with the finger so the rectum is cleaned and with this practice sensations take place in shakti nadi which awaken pingala nadi. After the awakening of pingala nadi, the pranas are awakened in the body; this awakening is called *pranotthana*. Thereafter, kundalini is awakened.

What is the correct environment for practising bahishkrita dhauti with water?

Swami Niranjanananda: This practice must be undertaken in a river where clean water is flowing. It cannot be done in a small amount of water, or in a well or reservoir where the water is stagnant. Therefore, given the state of the planet at present, it is not recommended that even qualified sadhakas attempt this practice. In the first place it would be extremely difficult to find a suitable water supply free from pollution. If such a place were found, it would be best to give thanks to one's *ishta devata*, or preferred form of God, and protect it, rather than polluting it with one's own bodily wastes.

When Sage Gheranda was teaching in India, rivers were still treated with great respect as *devis*, divine beings. Just as a child may be washed while sitting on its mother's lap, so a yogi would go to the river for self-purification. At that time, just a few centuries ago, people's everyday wastes were made use of in fertilizing the land, not completely misused by being poured into these streams of life that are so denigrated today.

MOOLA SHODHANA: ANAL CLEANSING

What is moola shodhana?

Swami Satyananda: The Sanskrit word *moola* literally means 'base' or 'root'. In this context, it means anus and rectum. The word *shodhana* means 'purification'. Therefore, *moola shodhana* can be translated as the practice which 'purifies the anus and rectum'.

This technique has various other common names. It is called *moola dhauti*, which means 'anal cleansing'. It is also called *ganesha kriya*. Ganesha is the name of the plump elephant deity of India, and the word *kriya* means 'action'. Therefore, this name can be translated as the 'elephant action'. Ganesha is closely connected with *mooladhara chakra*, the psychic centre near the region of the anus. This is one reason for the name Ganesha kriya. Also elephants wash themselves thoroughly with their trunk; possibly they also clean their anus in the same manner, at least externally. This practice is also called *chakrikarma*, which means the 'rotation practice'. It is so called because the finger is rotated within the anus and rectum.

Why is a turmeric root used in moola shodhana?

Swami Satyananda: Traditionally, a turmeric root is recommended for this practice. The turmeric plant is widely available in India and has great medicinal value as an antiseptic, blood purifier and general cleanser of physical impurities. It has astringent properties, which is the reason that it is used in moola shodhana. It tends to stimulate the nerves of the inside of the anus and rectum, which encourages bowel movement (peristalsis) and a free flow of blood. Thus it physically removes waste material and stimulates the natural function of the bowels.

Turmeric is not widely available in many countries, but one's finger can be used instead for moola shodhana. This is as good as turmeric, for though it is not astringent, there is more facility for manipulation.

How is moola shodhana performed?

Swami Niranjanananda: It is essential to sit in a squatting position for this practice. This position opens up the anus and the thighs exert pressure on the stomach, which helps move the faeces downwards.

A soft turmeric stem or the middle finger is used in moola shadhana. The turmeric stem should have the same dimensions as, and be no bigger than, the middle finger. The soft turmeric root should be cleaned properly and the outer layer peeled off so that its juice starts dripping.

The stem is gently inserted into the anus and kept inside for two or three minutes so that the juice of the peeled stem spreads inside the anus and rectum. One quality of turmeric is that it absorbs toxins; all toxic matter or wastes of the body are pulled towards the turmeric stem. After two or three minutes the stem is removed and disposed of.

If a turmeric root is not available, the middle finger can be used. Be sure the nail is clipped short. If the finger does not go in easily, contract the sphincter muscles and then release them, keeping the finger slightly inside. This will definitely help the process, but do not apply too much pressure. However far the finger goes in easily is sufficient. Traditionally ghee, clarified butter made from cow's milk, is applied to the finger. It is then inserted about four centimetres into the anus and rotated clockwise and anticlockwise so that the ghee is thoroughly applied. Pure ghee has many medicinal properties. The ghee should be homemade.

The finger is then removed, properly washed, ghee is applied and the finger is again inserted and rotated as before. This process can be repeated several times, but two or three minutes of practice are sufficient. In *Hatharatnavali* (1:28) it is written:

> *Paayunaale prasaaryaarddhaamanguleem bhraamayedabheeh.*
> *Yaavadgudavikaasassyaat chakrikarma nigadyate.*

> Half of the finger should be inserted in the anal canal, and moved around all the sides clockwise and anti-clockwise until the anus is fully stretched. This is called chakrikarma.

Should the muscles be contracted during moola shodhana?

Swami Satyananda: Moola shodhana can be intensified by alternately contracting and releasing the anal sphincter while the finger is inserted. This increases the stimulation of the nerves and the blood supply in the rectum, which in turn leads to improved health and functioning of this important part of the body.

When should moola shodhana be practised?

Swami Satyananda: This depends on one's personal circumstances. The stimulation induced by moola shodhana is sufficient to start off a chain reaction of peristalsis. Therefore, those who are constipated are advised to practise before trying to defecate.

Those who have a regular motion can try moola shodhana after passing stool. This will further stimulate the associated nerves and muscles and lead to the best possible evacuation and cleanliness of the anus and rectum. The best time is early in the morning.

When and how often should moola shodhana be practised?

Swami Niranjanananda: People suffering from constipation should do this practice first thing in the morning. Those who have regular bowel motions can practise moola shodhana after their morning ablutions. Morning is the ideal time for the practice. In order to rid the body of problems like piles, this practice should be done daily for at least a month.

How does moola shodhana work?

Swami Satyananda: Some knowledge of the anatomy of the area is helpful in understanding how moola shodhana works. There are two parts: the anus proper and the rectum. The anus is comprised of two sphincters, which can be dilated and contracted at will. These sphincter muscles seal the exit of the anus until the time of defecation. The anus is about two centimetres long, after which it merges with the rectum. The rectum continues upwards for a short distance to join the lower part of the descending colon.

If the finger is inserted one feels striations or projections. There are seven or eight of these, and they are about one centimetre in height. There are also valves in this area. There is a rich supply of nerves and blood vessels. It is these blood vessels that so easily distend to form haemorrhoids. This region is directly supplied by nerves from the sympathetic and the parasympathetic nervous systems.

Moola shodhana stimulates the nerves and blood vessels, enouraging the whole eliminative system to function efficiently. It also encourages regular and strain-free defecation and cleans the whole area of hard, encrusted and putrid waste matter. It removes and prevents ailments such as constipation and haemorrhoids (piles).

Moola shodhana can help change one's attitude towards life. The wonder of a regular free motion leads to a more relaxed disposition. It is such a simple practice, but it has far reaching effects.

Why should one practise moola shodhana?

Swami Niranjanananda: This practice is as useful as it is simple. The blood flow and the flow of energy through the nadis are increased, enabling the excretory system to function efficiently, and removing disorders, especially of the anus and rectum. Hardened faeces are expelled. Daily cleansing of the bowels with this technique changes a person's attitude towards life, as it provides relief from the misery of constipation. Once constipation is cured, many other diseases subside. All the systems of the body are affected by blockages in the rectum, so keeping this passage clean with the practice of moola shodhana improves the health in many ways.

The main physical purpose of practising moola shodhana is to relieve constipation. In constipation, the faeces may become as hard as stone, and the exertion needed to pass the stool causes pain and often damages the lining of the rectum and anus. Such straining can also cause haemorrhoids. Moola shodhana is an effective way of bringing relief. By applying ghee or turmeric juice inside the rectum, hardened faeces can be expelled with greater ease. The hardened kernels are to some extent broken up into smaller pieces as they are expelled and the rectum is lubricated, so injury to the anus is avoided.

However, moola shodhana should be adopted only when constipation has become severe and chronic and there is no other option. Practices such as laghoo shankhaprakshalana which help prevent this condition should also be regularly employed. In shankhaprakshalana the faeces are excreted after having been softened with water. Moola shodhana is the final practice of dhauti.

In *Hatharatnavali* (1:29) it is written:

Moolavyaadhirgulmarogo nashyatyatra mahodarah
Malashuddhirdeepanam cha jaayate chakrikarmanaa.

Piles, diseases of the spleen and distended stomach are cured; evacuation of the bowels, and stimulation of the digestive fire take place through chakrikarma.

What precautions should be taken when practising moola shodhana?

Swami Niranjanananda: The anal region and the skin inside are soft and delicate. If using turmeric, be sure it is fresh and soft. If turmeric is not available, the hands should be thoroughly washed before and after the practice, and ensure that the finger nails are trimmed properly.

People suffering from haemorrhoids or piles should be careful when inserting either the turmeric stem or the finger. When washing the finger or the anus during the practice, always be careful to use only cold water. Blood vessels contract on contact with cold water and dilate with hot water, increasing the blood flow. Using hot water will therefore exacerbate the swelling associated with piles.

What is the effect of moola shodhana on apana vayu?

Swami Niranjanananda: Moola shodhana is the last practice of the dhauti techniques. Its literal meaning is cleansing the root of the body. The root of the body is the rectum, so moola shodhana means cleaning the area of the rectum. In *Gheranda Samhita* (1:42–44) the effects of the practice are described:

Apaanakrooratаa taavadyaavanmoolam na shodhaye
Tasmaatsarvaprayatnena moolashodhanamaacharet.

Peetamoolasya dandena madhyamaangulinaa'pi vaa;
Yatnena kshaalayedguhyam vaarinaa cha punah punah.

Vaarayetkoshthakaathinyamaamaajeerna nivaarayet;
Kaaranam kaantipushtyoshcha deepanam vahnimandalam.

Cruel (disorders of) apana vayu cannot be removed without performing moola shodhana (anal cleansing). (42)

Cleaning of the anus is essential with a turmeric root or the middle finger combined with repeated washing with water. (43)

This practice removes hard faeces and constipation, the body becomes graceful and healthy and the digestive fire is stimulated. (44)

In verse 42, it is said, *apaana-kroorataa taavadyaavan-moolam na shodhayet*, as long as the root portion cannot be cleaned, apana vayu becomes cruel or ruthless, which means that disorders take place in apana vayu. Therefore, the function and importance of apana vayu needs to be understood.

First there is *maha prana*, the great prana that energizes the universe. Then there are the five prana vayus, which are subordinate manifestations of maha prana. These five prana vayus form the basis of yogic therapy. Sometimes they are simply called the five *vayus*, flows of energy, and sometimes they are called the five *pranas*, energies.

The five pranas regulate and coordinate the various organs and systems of the body. According to the science of yoga the practitioner can skilfully purify and work with these five pranas: prana, apana, samana, udana and vyana.

The second prana vayu is *apana*, which is downward flowing. It is situated in the pelvic region between the navel and perineum. Apana sustains the functions of the kidneys, bladder, bowels, excretory and reproductive organs, and is responsible for the expulsion of waste matter from the body, including gas, faeces and urine. The ejaculation of sperm, monthly cleansing of the womb and the expulsion of the foetus in childbirth are all part of the renewal work performed by apana vayu. A defect in its flow can result in disorders such as constipation or haemorrhoids, or the development of diseases in the kidneys and excretory system. Apana vayu is corrected by the practice of moola shodhana.

6

Danta Dhauti: Head Cleansing

What is danta dhauti?

Swami Satyananda: The ancient yogis realized the necessity of maintaining the sensory organs in optimum condition. *Danta dhauti*, one of the shatkarmas, consists of a series of simple practices which clean various organs and regions of the head. These practices are *danta moola dhauti*, cleaning of the teeth and gums, *jihva moola dhauti*, cleaning of the tongue, *kapala randhra dhauti*, washing the skull, *karna dhauti*, cleaning the ears and *chakshu dhauti*, washing the eyes.

These practices, as well as jala neti, are concerned either directly or indirectly with four senses of the body – hearing, seeing, smelling and tasting. As such they are important in enabling us to gain the best possible perception of the world around us. Our sensory perceptions are dependent on the state of the associated organs. Therefore, the practices of danta dhauti, though perhaps seeming rather trivial and simple, are a valuable aid to being able to clearly communicate with and relate to the outside world.

Why does hatha yoga include danta dhauti?

Swami Niranjanananda: The literal meaning of *danta dhauti* is cleaning the teeth, but here it means cleaning and purifying the region of the head. The first practice is *dantamoolam*, cleaning the teeth and gums. The second practice is *jihvaamoolam*, cleaning the tongue and its root. *Randhram cha karnayugmayoh* means cleaning the two ear orifices – the left and right ears are cleaned separately, so it is considered to be two dhautis. *Kapaalarandhra* means cleaning the upper portion of the frontal part of the head. These are the five types of danta dhauti. They are listed in *Gheranda Samhita* (1:25):

> *Dantamoolam jihvaamoolam randhram cha karnayugmayoh;*
> *Kapaalarandhra panchaite dantadhautirvidheeyate.*
>
> There are five kinds of danta dhauti: dantamoola (cleaning the teeth), jihvamoola (cleaning the tongue), karnarandhra (cleaning the two ears) and kapalarandhra (cleaning the upper region of the head). Thus there are five in all.

These practices are used for complete purification of four *jnanendriyas*, organs of sensory knowledge: ears, eyes, tongue and nose plus the teeth. It is the first duty of a yoga aspirant to clean the skin, teeth, mouth, tongue, ears and nose every morning. Knowledge of the world around one comes through the jnanendriyas, so if they are not kept clean, the perception will be defective. Maximum significance has been given to cleansing these sense organs.

DANTAMOOLA DHAUTI: CLEANING THE TEETH

What is dantamoola dhauti?

Swami Satyananda: The Sanskrit word *danta* means 'teeth', *dhauti* means 'wash' and *moola* means 'root'. Therefore this practice is concerned with cleaning the teeth and gums.

What items are used to clean the teeth?

Swami Satyananda: The usual utensil used today is the toothbrush. Unfortunately toothbrush bristles can become a breeding ground for germs and bacteria. During daily use these are transmitted into the mouth. Furthermore, hard bristles tend to tear and damage the gums, especially when the cleaning action is harsh.

In India, the traditional method of cleaning the teeth is by means of a twig from a neem tree. The twig is usually about fifteen centimetres long and half a centimetre thick, and it has good alkaline and astringent properties. The end of the stick is chewed until it forms bristles. These are then used to brush the teeth and gums. Both chewing the end of the stick and using it as a brush makes the teeth and gums strong and clean. After use the stick is thrown away. This method, however, is probably impractical for most people. If this is the case, use a soft-bristled brush to clean the teeth and try to clean the brush as often as possible.

The gums should be cleaned by using the index finger to make a hard, rubbing motion over both the inner and outer gums. The teeth should be cleaned at least twice a day, and preferably after each meal.

The important qualities of a dentifrice are that it is sufficiently abrasive to remove ingrained stains on the teeth, germicidal to destroy bacteria, as well as being able to wash the teeth and gums. The ancient yogis always made their own tooth powder out of Acacia catechu, alum, and the ash of burnt coconut shells. However, these substances are not readily available and so most people have to use the toothpastes of today.

What are the basic guidelines for maintaining healthy teeth and gums?

Swami Satyananda: The importance of maintaining healthy gums and teeth is not appreciated by many people. The mouth is the gateway to the body and a favourite breeding ground for bacteria. Some of these germs make their way further into the body while many remain in food particles trapped in the teeth cavities. The vulnerable time for tooth decay and the build up of bacteria in the teeth and gums is in the first half an hour or so after meals. It is for this reason that the teeth and gums should be cleaned immediately after each meal.

Diet also has a large part to play in the health of the teeth and gums. This is illustrated by the fact that there are many cases of primitive tribes who have perfect sets of teeth, yet have never seen a toothbrush in their life. Diets which are rich in sugar have a deleterious influence on teeth and gums, as sugary foods are quickly converted into acids, which in turn attack the enamel or protective lining of the teeth.

Regular cleaning of the teeth and gums, together with a reduction in the intake of sugary food and the adoption of a sensible vitamin-rich diet is therefore the only sure way to prevent dental decay and pyorrhoea, as well as the accompanying toothache and bad breath. It is also believed that unhealthy teeth and gums, and infections of this area, have a harmful influence on the general health of the whole body.

Why does dantamoola dhauti emphasize cleaning the gums as well as the teeth?

Swami Niranjanananda: The modern method of using a toothbrush cleans the teeth, but not the gums. The gums are extremely important as they provide the foundation for the teeth. After brushing the teeth, the gums must be massaged with a finger for two to four minutes. In *Gheranda Samhita* (1:26–27) it is written:

Khaadirena rasenaatha shuddhamrittikayaa tathaa;
Maarjayeddantamoolam cha yaavatkilvishamaaharet.

Dantamoolam paraadhautiryoginaam yoga saadhane;
Nityam kuryaatprabhaate cha dantarakshaa cha yogavit;
Dantamoolam dhaavanaadikaaryeshu yoginaam matam.

Rub or massage the roots of the teeth with the juice of the khadira plant (Acacia catechu) or with clean earth until the impurities are removed. (26)

Yogis must adopt this method every morning to protect their teeth. Those who know yoga consider dantamoola dhauti to be a significant part of the purification process. (27)

Sage Gheranda emphasizes that cleaning the roots of the teeth removes dirt and disorders and maintains healthy gums. Generally, people are particular about diet and clothes, but often become careless about the mouth, and think that cleaning the teeth only means removing the surface dirt. Yogis take care of their teeth with the practice of dantamoola.

What is the traditional hatha yoga method for cleaning the teeth and gums?

Swami Niranjanananda: A special medicine prepared from the leaves of the khadira or Acacia catechu plant is used. Soak the catechu leaves, put the juice on a finger and rub it on the roots of the teeth. Catechu is a medicinal plant used in ayurveda. If there is swelling in the gums, blisters in the mouth, toothache, cavities or bacteria, sucking catechu is suggested. Catechu has been in use from earliest times to protect and strengthen the teeth.

If catechu is not available, pure black or yellow clay dug out of wet soil can also be used. Ensure that it contains no small pieces of stone. The clay is made into a paste and rubbed on the roots of the gums for two to three minutes, followed by gargling. This is repeated five or six times.

The catechu should be made into a fine powder, otherwise it can scratch the gums. Anyone who suffers from gum disease or dental caries should only undertake this practice after appropriate dental treatment.

What are the benefits of healthy gums and teeth?

Swami Niranjanananda: The practice of dantamoola dhauti maintains healthy gums and a strong blood flow. It is well known that food particles collect between the teeth and produce bacteria and other germs which are harmful not only for the teeth, but also for the health of the body. After some time the effect of dental disorders is seen in one's overall health. If there is bleeding from the gums, pyorrhoea, blisters or ulcers in the mouth, blood or pus entering the body from the mouth affects the digestive system and also other systems of the body. For example, dental decay can occasionally affect the heart. Premature loss of teeth is due to lack of proper care. Hence, Sage Gheranda has mentioned cleanliness of the teeth and gums.

According to yogis the gums should be massaged both inside and outside at least three times a day. This exerts pressure on the roots of the teeth and gums from both sides, improving the blood flow to the cells.

JIHVA SHODHANA: CLEANING THE TONGUE

What is the purpose of jihva shodhana?

Swami Satyananda: The Sanskrit word *jihva* means 'tongue' and *moola* means 'root'. This practice is therefore concerned with cleaning the tongue and its root.

The tongue is a vital organ of the body, yet few people ever seriously think about cleaning it. Everyone has at some time noticed a thick layer of yellow slime on the upper surface of the tongue, especially first thing in the morning and when feeling a little unwell. This coating on the tongue actually consists of impurities that have been removed from the body. It indicates that there is some inner disorder or accumulation of toxins that the body is desperately trying to expel.

Failure to remove the impurities on the tongue can aggravate ailments within the body, particularly digestive problems. These impurities can act as breeding grounds for bacteria which can in turn contaminate food being eaten. Therefore, regular cleaning of the tongue is important in maintaining a healthy body. The practice is simple and takes no more than a minute or so.

Why is jihva shodhana important?

Swami Niranjanananda: The practice of *jihva shodhana* or *jihvamoola dhauti* involves cleaning and massaging the tongue. Through this practice the length of the tongue is increased and health is optimized. Many kinds of chemical reactions take place in the body. New cells are generated, old ones die and waste material is expelled. The coating that develops on the tongue is cellular debris and micro-organisms which are not needed by the body. It is recommended that these impurities be removed daily by the practice of jihva dhauti. In *Gheranda Samhita* (1:28) it is written:

Athaatah sampravakshyaami jihvaashodhana kaaranam;
Jaraamaranarogaadeennaashayeddeerghalambikaa.

Now I will tell you the method for cleaning the tongue. Lengthening of the tongue destroys old age, death and disease.

How is jihva shodhana performed?

Swami Niranjanananda: Butter is applied to the tongue. The index, middle and ring fingers are then carefully inserted into the throat and the root of the tongue is massaged for some time. A milking action is then performed by holding the sides of the tongue with the thumb and fingers. The butter makes the tongue slippery and the milking action becomes easy. This practice should be done seven to ten times every morning and evening. It is described in *Gheranda Samhita* (1:29–31):

Tarjaneemadhyamaanaamaa angulitrayayogatah;
Veshayedgalamadhye tu maarjayellambikaamoolam;
Shanaih shanaih maarjayitvaa kaphadosham nivaarayet.

Maarjayennavaneetena dohayechcha punah punah;
Tadagram lohayantrena karshayitvaa shanaih shanaih.

Nityam kuryaatprayatnena raverudayake'stake;
Evam krite cha nityam saa lambikaa deerghataam vrajet.

The root of the tongue should be cleaned by inserting the index finger, middle finger and ring finger in the throat. Kapha disorders (phlegm) are removed by slowly and gently rubbing the tongue. (29)

Once this cleaning and rubbing is over, apply a little butter on the tongue. Again perform the action like that of milking a cow. Thereafter, stretch the tongue out with the help of small tongs. (30)

The length of the tongue increases by doing this practice daily at the time of sunrise and sunset. (31)

When should jihva shodhana be performed?

Swami Satyananda: This practice should preferably be performed before breakfast. This is important as otherwise one may retch as the fingers are pushed into the back of the throat.

Try to practise at least once daily, if not twice a day. Two minutes rubbing the back of tongue and two minutes milking the upper and lower surfaces is sufficient.

What precautions should be taken when practising jihva shodhana?

Swami Niranjanananda: The practice is to be done gently, especially if there are ulcers on the tongue. The fingernails should be closely trimmed. Do not force the fingers in too deeply as this may hurt or injure the larynx.

Why is jihva shodhana an important yogic practice?

Swami Niranjanananda: The tongue has important sensory and motor functions. As it is richly supplied with nerves, there is a particularly strong connection with the brain. According to yoga, if the tongue is diseased, the thinking becomes dull and the breathing process may also be impaired. Therefore, proper care and maintenance of the tongue is necessary. By massaging the tongue with a milking motion, the mucus that collects in the throat and windpipe is cleared. This massage is the best means of cleaning the tongue.

A long tongue is considered more useful for speech. Speech disorders can occur due to a short tongue. In order to lengthen it, after milking, the tongue is slowly stretched out and held with a pair of clean iron tongs or if small tongs are not available, the tongue can be held between the thumb and fingers for two to three minutes. This practice makes the muscles of the tongue flexible. Daily practice lengthens the tongue. It is said that the tongue of a yoga practitioner should be so long that it touches *bhrumadhya*, the eyebrow centre, or at least the end of the nose.

KARNARANDHRA DHAUTI: CLEANING THE EARS

What is karnarandhra dhauti?

Swami Satyananda: The word *karna* means 'ear', and this practice is concerned with cleaning the ears.

What is the structure of the ear canal?

Swami Satyananda: The outer portion of the ear consists of a short tube or canal about four centimetres in length, running from the outside to the inside of the head. Inside the tube there are a few hairs which prevent insects and other foreign bodies from entering the inner regions of the head and the eardrum at the end of the canal. This outer canal also contains various glands, which secrete wax to protect the deeper structures of the ear.

How important is cleanliness of the ear canal for hearing?

Swami Satyananda: For perfect hearing, the outer canal must be clear so that the sound vibrations in the air can cause the ear to vibrate. Sometimes the glands produce too much wax which blocks the canal; or sometimes wax accumulates, even though it is produced in correct amounts. This can reduce one's hearing capacity.

What methods are used to clean the ears?

Swami Satyananda: A varied assortment of methods and utensils are used to clean the ears. Some people even use toothpicks or matchsticks. These devices are not advised as they can easily damage the eardrums. The best method is to gently place the small finger in the ear canal and rotate the finger a number of times. A slight pressure should be applied against the ear walls to dislodge any unnecessary wax. Remove the finger and direct the head and ear canal downwards to allow any dry wax to drop out. Repeat the same procedure but use the index finger. There should be a layer of wax on the fingers after completing the practice. Repeat with the other ear.

Perform this practice every week or so, ensuring that the fingernails are short and clean.

How should the ears be cleaned?

Swami Niranjanananda: There are many modern methods of cleaning the ear canals. Many companies sell cotton buds (cotton on the end of a plastic stick). According to yoga, however, cleansing should be done with a finger. Plastic sticks and matchsticks are very thin. According to yoga and modern medicine, it is both unnecessary and potentially harmful to stick such objects into the ears. If they go deep inside by mistake, the ear drum can be damaged. A finger, however, will not go in deep enough to cause such damage.

There are two techniques for karnarandhra dhauti. In the first technique either the index or ring finger is used. The finger is wet so that it adheres to the skin at the mouth of the ear canal. Next, the finger is slowly inserted with pressure into the inside of the ear and rotated. When practised correctly, a vacuum-like effect is created so that suction takes place and gently starts pulling out the dirt and wax from inside. This is the practice recommended by Sage Gheranda. In *Gheranda Samhita* (1:32) this technique is described:

> *Tarjanyanaamika yogaanmaarjayetkarnarandhrayoh;*
> *Nityamabhyaasa yogena naadaantaram prakaashayet.*

> Clean the orifices of both ears with the index and ring fingers. By practising this daily, nada or inner sound may be heard.

An alternative technique is to boil two pieces of garlic in sesame oil or any other pure edible oil. Traditionally, a piece of cotton wool or the end of a finger was dipped in the oil so that the oil could drip, drop by drop, into the ear. Today a sterile ear dropper bought from a chemist can be used. Let the oil drip into the ear, carefully putting only two to four drops in each ear. Any dirt and wax will swell up and is easily removed by cleaning with the finger.

What are the benefits of karnarandhra dhauti?

Swami Niranjanananda: Wax collects continuously inside the ear tubes. If the ears are not cleaned regularly, pieces of dirt accumulate and block the ears. According to yogis, when the ring or index finger is put inside the ear and moved briskly, dirt and wax stick to the finger and are removed.

Also, by briskly rotating the finger, the blood flow within the ear is enhanced, which cannot be achieved with a stick. This increased blood flow may help prevent ear diseases. Part of the skin of the ears is connected to the parasympathetic vagus nerve, the stimulation of which relaxes certain internal organs – for example, it slows the heart rate. With this process balance is achieved in the autonomic nervous system.

Sometimes excessive wax is produced, blocking the ear canal, which can cause hearing difficulties. In such conditions, doctors may rinse the ears with water, pushing warm water into the ear canal with a syringe, to soften and flush out the wax.

How can cleaning the ears assist the practice of nada yoga?

Swami Niranjanananda: Nada yoga is an independent branch of yoga. *Nada yoga* means hearing the internal sound in a state of *dharana*, concentration, and *dhyana*, meditation. According to nada yoga, the hearing sense not only catches external sounds, but also subtle sounds that are created inside. When a person progresses in sadhana and attains the state of dharana or dhyana, one enters into new depths of consciousness by catching hold of those subtle internal sounds with awareness. This is one technique of nada yoga. In the absence of strong hearing, however, subtle sounds cannot be heard. When the ears remain clean, the hearing capacity is enhanced and slowly, with regular practice, the practitioner becomes capable of listening to the internal *nada*. In the practice of nada yoga, one first listens to the physical sounds created inside the body, like the sounds of the breath, blood circulation, heartbeat, etc. While listening to them, a state of consciousness is reached where different sounds start to be heard. Sometimes the sound of a bell is heard, sometimes the sound of a conch, a flute, or a waterfall. These subtle sounds keep on changing. Beyond gross sound, in the subtle state itself, extremely subtle sounds can be heard. As one-pointedness increases and one goes deep inside, nada like the sound of the vibration in an atom can be heard.

This is the practice of nada yoga. Karnarandhra dhauti, cleaning the ears, is a practical aid to making consciousness subtle so that nada is heard.

CHAKSHU DHAUTI: CLEANING THE EYES

What is chakshu dhauti?

Swami Satyananda: This practice involves washing the eyes with clean, lukewarm water whenever time permits. This can be done when taking a wash or bath, making sure that no soap enters the eyes.

KAPALARANDHRA DHAUTI: CLEANING THE UPPER HEAD

What is kapalarandhra dhauti?

Swami Satyananda: Kapalarandhra is the upper, slightly hollow region of the head, which can be clearly seen on a newborn baby. Therefore, kapalarandhra dhauti is concerned with washing the upper part of the head. The practices are simple and require little description.

The first technique is to wash the head vigorously and thoroughly with cold water. This has a soothing influence on the whole brain, and is useful when one feels tired or sluggish, as it instantly brings wakefulness and vitality.

Another technique of kapalarandhra is kapala dhauti. One presses the temples on each side of the forehead with the thumbs, making small circling movements. Do this for a minute or so, then repeat the same movement rotating the thumbs in the opposite direction. This brings relaxation to the brain and is especially useful if one has a headache.

How is kapalarandhra dhauti practised and what are its benefits?

Swami Niranjanananda: There are several practices of *kapalarandhra,* cleaning the openings in the skull. In *Gheranda Samhita* (1:33) *bhalarandhra* is mentioned – this is usually interpreted to mean the forehead or the depression just above the eyebrow centre. Sage Gheranda recommends this practice to stimulate the 'third eye' of insight. This relates to the faculty of *divya drishti,* divine vision, which is associated with ajna chakra.

Another practice of kapalarandhra, also dealing with the spiritual nature, relates to sahasrara chakra and *brahmarandhra,* the opening to higher consciousness, at the crown of the head. Brahmarandhra, which is sometimes called kapalarandhra, is a door. If this part of the skull is observed in a newborn baby, a small depression or even a pulse beat against the skin will be noticed. There is an opening called the fontanelle, which closes as a child grows up. This region is associated with the cerebral cortex, which is responsible for many higher functions, including speech and decision making.

The fontanelle is in the region of sahasrara. When real yogis release prana from their bodies, they do so consciously. When a yogi does not want rebirth on earth, the prana is released from this exit only, i.e. from sahasrara chakra. It means that the life force enters and leaves the body at brahmarandhra.

The technique given in *Gheranda Samhita* is simple and straightforward, but has long-lasting, subtle benefits. As a regular practice, on first waking, after meals and before sleeping, one should consciously relax. With the forehead relaxed, and preferably with the eyes closed, lightly massage the part of the forehead just above the nose with the right thumb. In *Gheranda Samhita* (1:33–34) the practice is described:

> *Vriddhangushthena dakshena maarjayedbhaalarandhrakam;*
> *Evamabhyaasayogena kaphadosham nivaarayet.*
>
> *Nadee nirmalataam yaati divyadrishtih prajaayate;*
> *Nidraante bhojanaante cha divaante cha dine dine.*
>
> Massage the forehead with the right hand thumb. With this type of practice one is relieved of kapha dosha. (33)
>
> The nadis are purified and divine vision is attained. Practise daily at the end of sleep, after food and before sleep. (34)

The light pressure and stimulation helps release mucous blockages from the nasal cavity and related sinuses, balancing kapha. It also helps one to centre, to relax further, and to be aware of one's subtle nature, awakening divya drishti. According to Sage Gheranda this practice cools the brain and is useful for cataracts and other eye disorders. Additionally, it is said to lower high blood pressure and protect against colds and coughs.

Another highly beneficial technique of kapalarandhra employs the cooling quality of water. Joining the fingers and thumb of the right hand, make a cup-like shape with the palm. Take water in the palm, lean forward and pat the upper portion of the head with the palm three or four times, so that the brahmarandhra becomes wet. Repeat this process four or five times.

This should be practised on waking, after the midday meal and in the evening. One point should be clarified.

If there is hair on the head, the water does not reach the skin unless the hair gets completely wet. Hair creates an obstruction to this practice. If it is not possible to practise three times a day, practise at least at the time of bathing.

Kapalarandhra dhauti provides coolness and calmness to the brain, so that freshness and creativity are experienced. This practice is most helpful during the hot summer season. The aim of this dhauti kriya is not only cleansing but also to provide coolness in brahmarandhra, as if this part of the body remains cool, alertness, mental agility and freshness are experienced. Washing the head makes one feel good: simply pouring water over the head makes one feel fresh, whether it is summer or winter.

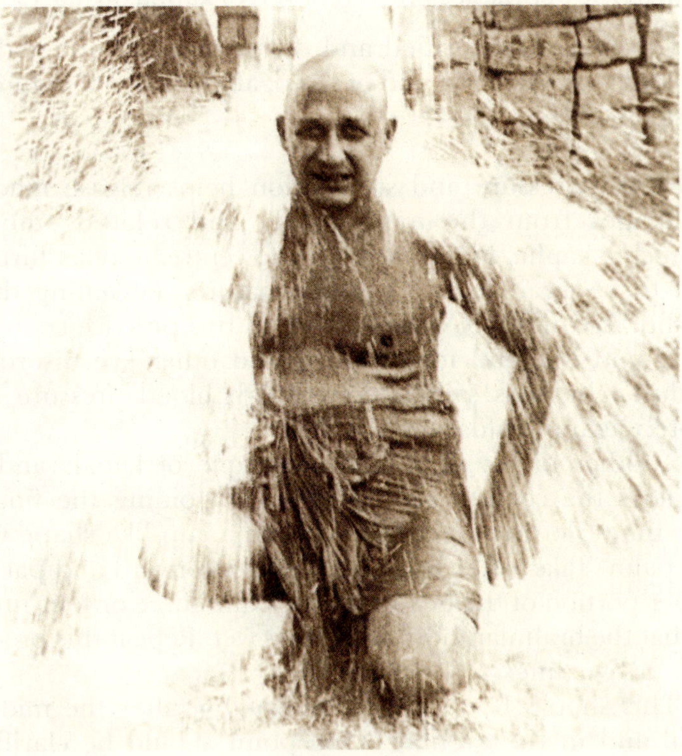

7

Hrid Dhauti: Cleansing the Heart Region

What is hrid dhauti?

Swami Niranjanananda: *Hrid* means heart, *dhauti* means cleanliness. The heart region here includes the oesophagus, lungs and stomach. Cleansing the oesophagus is easy, even cleaning the stomach is simple, but cleaning the lungs is more complex. These practices are grouped under the heading of *hrid dhauti.*

The practice of hrid dhauti can be done in three ways. The first type is *danda dhauti,* which uses a *danda*, a stick made from sugarcane, the stem of a banana tree, or a thin turmeric root. The second type is *vaman dhauti,* using water. The third type is *vastra dhauti,* which uses *vastra*, a piece of cloth.

These methods of hrid dhauti work by creating a vacuum in the chest so that kapha and impurities collected inside the lungs and windpipe can be expelled. They are listed in *Gheranda Samhita* (1:35):

> *Hriddhautim trividhaam kuryaaddandavamanavaasasaa.*
>
> There are three types of hrid dhauti: using a stick, regurgitating water, and using cloth.

Hrid dhauti, therefore, has these three practices. The first practice is danda dhauti, which is difficult, secret and not applicable to all. The second practice is vaman dhauti, which is of two types: jala vaman and anna vaman, known respectively as kunjal and vyaghra kriya. The third type of hrid dhauti is vastra dhauti, which is difficult but especially beneficial for the body.

DANDA DHAUTI: CLEANING WITH A STICK

What is danda dhauti?

Swami Niranjanananda: Danda dhauti is a difficult practice, performed by inserting a specially prepared stick into the throat. As is seen in circus performances, some people can insert a sword into the throat. Similarly, a hatha yogi inserts the stem, and keeps holding it. In order to do this practice, breath retention must first be perfected. As long as one is breathing in and out, this practice cannot be done, as the throat and windpipe will be moving. The rod is inserted only while retaining the breath. Danda dhauti is described in *Gheranda Samhita* (1:36–37):

> *Rambhaadandam hariddandam vetradandam tathaiva cha;*
> *Hrinmadhye chaalayitvaa tu punah pratyaaharechchhanaih.*
>
> *Kapham pittam tathaa kledam rechayedoordhvavartmanaa;*
> *Dandadhautividhaanena hridrogam naashayed dhruvam.*
>
> The stem of a soft portion of the banana tree, a thin turmeric stem or a sugarcane stem should be repeatedly inserted (through the mouth) and then slowly withdrawn from the middle chest. (36)
>
> Then kapha, pitta and mucus should be evacuated through the mouth. This practice definitely destroys even heart disease. (37)

Danda dhauti is not suitable for everyone and should not be practised by anyone without expert personal guidance. A much safer form of hrid dhauti is vaman dhauti.

Why is danda dhauti practised?

Swami Niranjanananda: The inner walls of the food pipe are covered with *kapha*, mucus, and *pitta*, bile. When this matter accumulates, it can enter the larynx and affect the respiratory system, reducing the breathing capacity, and producing a wheezing sound while inhaling. With danda dhauti, kapha and pitta are expelled with *rechaka kriya*, exhalation.

VAMAN DHAUTI: CLEANSING WITH REGURGITATION

What is vaman dhauti?

Swami Satyananda: *Vaman dhauti* is cleaning the digestive tract from the stomach to the mouth by means of vomiting. Both *kunjal* and *vaman* mean 'vomiting'; *kriya* means 'practice' and *dhauti* means 'wash'.

There are generally three ways vaman dhauti can be done. In *kunjal kriya* water is drunk on an empty stomach and regurgitated by rubbing the back of the tongue. In *vyaghra kriya* water is drunk three to four hours after eating and the contents of the stomach are then regurgitated. In *gaja karani*, water is drunk on an empty stomach and regurgitated by contracting the upper abdomen while simultaneously inhaling.

What are the different types of vaman dhauti?

Swami Niranjanananda: The most commonly practised types of vaman dhauti are kunjal kriya and vyaghra kriya. Kunjal kriya is done on an empty stomach and vyaghra kriya is done after meals. Kunjal kriya is done when one feels normal and healthy, whereas vyaghra kriya should be practised when there is a disorder or discomfort in the stomach.

KUNJAL KRIYA: WATER REGURGITATION

How is kunjal kriya performed?

Swami Satyananda: To perform kunjal kriya at least six glasses of saline water are drunk in quick succession,

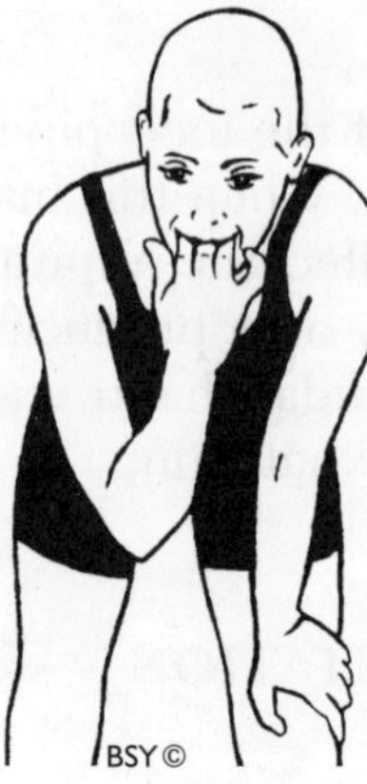

Kunjal kriya

until the stomach cannot hold anymore. It is most important to drink quickly and not just sip the water. When the stomach is full, the urge to vomit occurs automatically. Leaning forward, one then opens the mouth and places the middle and index fingers of the right hand as far back on the tongue as possible. The tongue is gently rubbed and pressed, inducing the water to gush out from the stomach. During the expulsion of water the fingers may be removed from the mouth, although this is not necessary. When the flow of water ceases, the back of the tongue is again pressed and the process repeated until the stomach is empty.

How can fear of vomiting be overcome when practising kunjal?

Swami Satyananda: This practice may seem a little repulsive to some people, but in reality kunjal kriya is a simple practice and all that is vomited is salty water containing impurities from the stomach. As such there is no unpleasant taste, smell or nausea as there is during times of sickness. It is these uncomfortable sensations that people find repulsive. Without these disagreeable factors the practice of kunjal kriya becomes simple and is not at all unpleasant. The biggest obstacle in trying this practice is the mental concept of what is involved.

How can vomiting be beneficial to health?

Swami Satyananda: Vomiting is normally the last resort of the stomach to throw out impure, excessively rich or heavy food. It is a natural physical process but only as a last resort. To purposely vomit is in a sense unnatural, but experience has shown that it is an effective way to improve the functioning of the stomach and in turn the whole physical body.

If the stomach was treated with more care it would not be necessary to do kunjal kriya, but sadly, most people mistreat their stomachs. It is under these circumstances that intentional vomiting becomes most useful as a means of removing the impurities that contaminate the body.

Who should practise vaman dhauti?

Swami Satyananda: The stomach should be kept clean and in the healthiest possible condition if it is to retain its efficiency and remain free from disease. Kunjal kriya creates this clean, healthy condition, as well as removing acidity. It is therefore a panacea for both those who have digestive ailments and those who want to maintain good health.

Vaman dhauti is especially beneficial for anyone suffering from asthma, bronchitis and acidity. Those who want to practise meditation but find their progress interrupted by acidity should use this practice.

What are the health benefits of practising kunjal kriya?

Swami Niranjanananda: Kunjal kriya helps a healthy person to remain free from disease. It cleans the upper digestive tract, has a profound effect on the nervous system, and is therefore beneficial for general health. It is especially useful for people suffering from kapha and pitta disorders.

Kunjal washes the digestive system from stomach to mouth, helping remove and prevent diseases caused by the accumulation of toxic matter and general impurities in this region. It helps eradicate bad breath, phlegm in the throat and some types of sore throat. Salty water reduces the secretion of acid by the glands in the stomach, enhancing the stomach's digestive efficacy.

Asthmatics obtain great relief from this practice. Kunjal can be practised at the time of an asthma attack. In this situation it is imperative that the stomach is completely filled with water to obtain best results. When the person starts vomiting, the airways, which are tight and contracted in an asthma attack are relaxed, providing immediate relief.

Why is kunjal so effective at relieving stomach problems?

Swami Satyananda: There are various causes of stomach problems – eating too much food, eating food that is too rich, bad or impure, as well as excess secretion of gastric juices, particularly acid, due to emotional upsets or sustained stress.

Kunjal cannot change one's food habits or remove mental and emotional tension. It can, however, help to keep the stomach in good order by washing it clean of impurities. The salt water also reduces the secretion of acid from the glands in the stomach. These glands become more efficient with the practice of kunjal, improving digestion. All these effects help prevent indigestion and allow the best possible assimilation of nutrients, as well as eliminating other digestive ailments. Whenever one feels a little queasy in the stomach, perhaps early in the morning, kunjal is recommended to bring relief.

There is another reason that kunjal is so beneficial. There is a tendency for the residue of undigested food to lie in the bottom of the stomach once all the easily digested food has passed into the intestines. This is particularly so if one has a distended stomach, for the bottom of the stomach is more than likely below the level of the outlet to the intestines (pyloric valve). This acts as a reservoir in which fermentation takes place. When the next meal is eaten this residue mixes with incoming food and can pass into the intestines, possibly contaminating and poisoning the system, as much of it will be absorbed into the bloodstream from the intestines. Kunjal kriya throws this fermented waste out of the stomach before it can cause harm. As such kunjal is a sure way of preventing auto-poisoning of the body.

Kunjal gives relief from biliousness. If the expelled water is green, it indicates the presence of bile. The bile is secreted from the gall bladder into the intestines below the stomach, but often finds its way up into the stomach, especially if it is oversecreted. Kunjal brings wonderful relief by eliminating the accumulation of this nauseating and bitter tasting bile.

Why does kunjal relieve asthma?

Swami Satyananda: Asthmatics find kunjal an excellent practice. Although there is no obvious connection between the lungs and the stomach, for a number of reasons, kunjal does bring relief. This is confirmed by the large blobs of phlegm which are thrown out by asthmatics during kunjal.

The warmth and salinity of the water thins the mucus, making it easier to expel. There is also stimulation of the sympathetic nervous system, causing the bronchii to become wider. This allows mucus to come out and air to come in. With the removal of blockages in the respiratory passages, kunjal brings great relief to the asthma sufferer by allowing easier breathing.

People who suffer from asthma can and should perform kunjal when they are actually having an attack as it terminates the spasm. In this case it is essential that the stomach is completely filled with water to obtain the best results. Though it may be difficult to drink the water down quickly due to shortage of breath, one must try; with determination it can be accomplished. The urge to vomit should be resisted, so that the stomach can be filled to the brim – bloated in fact. The bronchial tubes, which tighten and contract during an attack of asthma, relax as soon as the water is expelled. This brings much needed and instant relief.

When and how often should kunjal be performed?

Swami Satyananda: Bearing in mind the capacity of the body and the person's health, kunjal should be undertaken only once a week unless an experienced yoga teacher advises otherwise.

The time of practice depends on the prevailing climate. It should not be done outside if the weather is cold. If practised indoors in a reasonably warm home, the outside weather has little influence and kunjal can be performed regardless of the climate.

The best time to practise kunjal is early in the morning, before breakfast. However, if the atmosphere is cold both inside and outside, it can be practised later in the day when it becomes warmer. Food should not be taken for at least half an hour after completing the practice. This allows time for the stomach lining to be re-established.

Normally this kriya should not be done after meals, allowing the stomach to perform its duties and empty itself of its contents. This process takes at least four hours depending on how much food is eaten, and if kunjal is practised prematurely, the food will be vomited. There is a similar technique called vyaghra kriya, which does this purposely but it is used during specific circumstances.

What are the obstacles to practising kunjal?

Swami Satyananda: The biggest hurdle to overcome with this practice is the disgust attached to the idea of vomiting. When first attempting kunjal, a little willpower must be used to carry it out to the full. It is easy to drink only one glass and persuade oneself that the stomach is now full; or to make plans to do the practice and then postpone it at the last moment until another day under the guise of some suitable excuse. But when one becomes accustomed to the idea and has tried it a few times it is no more difficult than cleaning the teeth and does not take much more time.

Who should not practise kunjal?

Swami Satyananda: Most people can do kunjal. However, it should not be attempted by those suffering from hernia of the stomach or abdomen, high blood pressure or heart problems.

Though kunjal kriya helps to remove excess acidity from the stomach, a factor associated with ulcers, it is not advisable to do this practice when there is excess acidity, as it may do more harm than good.

If there are any doubts about whether or not to do kunjal kriya, the guidance of a competent yoga teacher must be sought.

Why is salt added to the water?
Swami Satyananda: The water can be either with or without salt. This is the practitioner's choice. The deciding factor depends on why the practice is being done. Salt water inhibits the secretion of acid in the stomach. For other purposes both unsalted and salted are suitable. If salt is added to the water, a reasonable proportion is one teaspoonful per litre of water.

Is salt the only suitable additive for kunjal water?
Swami Satyananda: Many people ask about using other herbs in place of salt. In ayurveda many other ingredients are used, but following the hatha yoga methods directly, salt is used, and it is the most harmless. The majority of people are unable to control the functions of the body and they do not know how weak or strong their body is. Therefore it is best to practise only with salt.

What temperature should the water be for kunjal?
Swami Satyananda: Lukewarm water is recommended, about body temperature. However, this is flexible. Water can be taken directly from the tap but it should not be too cold. This is important as during the practice the stomach will be filled with a large volume of water; if it is too cold it could easily chill the body. Needless to say, the water should be clean.

How important is it to drink all the water?
Swami Satyananda: The maximum quantity of water should be drunk, even if it seems beyond one's capacity. The water should gush out of the mouth in full force. All the water must be vomited out.

What should be done if regurgitation doesn't occur?
Swami Satyananda: Many teachers say that the best way to induce expulsion of water is to touch the uvula (the small pendant hanging from the soft palate above the root of the tongue). This is not advisable as it tends to cause retching

and not a smooth elimination of water. It is preferable to press the root of the tongue. If the water still doesn't come up, don't worry. Though the benefits of kunjal will be lost, it will not cause any harm. The water will merely pass through the system in the normal way. It may give a looser than normal bowel motion, but for those who suffer from constipation this is not such a bad result.

What are the contra-indications for the practice of kunjal?
Swami Niranjanananda: Kunjal increases blood pressure so it should not be attempted by people suffering from high blood pressure. People suffering from peptic ulcers, hernia, raised intracranial pressure, diabetes with eye problems or any kind of heart disease should not do this practice. Though kunjal kriya removes hyperacidity from the stomach, practising it for hyperacidity is not recommended as the risk of harm outweighs the potential benefits. It is not recommended during pregnancy.

Kunjal should not be attempted without direct guidance, as problems can occur.

What effect does kunjal have on the emotions?
Swami Niranjanananda: Kunjal kriya is an exceptionally effective technique for relieving pent-up, unexpressed emotions which burden the heart and cause feelings of heaviness within the body and mind, particularly around the chest, diaphragm and abdomen. The technique is especially useful for releasing emotional blocks created by inner and external tension, conflict and pressure. It brings about a feeling of emotional lightness, clarity and peace, which in turn supports one's physical health.

VYAGHRA KRIYA: TIGER PRACTICE

What is vyaghra kriya?
Swami Satyananda: Vaman dhauti or *vyaghra kriya* is the second practice of hrid dhauti. Vaman is 'to vomit', vyaghra

is 'tiger'. In this practice the food from the stomach is vomited three hours after a meal. This practice is also called *baghi kriya*. Both *vyaghra* and *baghi* mean 'tiger'. This technique is therefore known as the tiger action of regurgitation. It is a similar practice to kunjal but a large portion of semi-digested food as well as water is expelled from the stomach.

Why is vyaghra kriya named after the tiger?

Swami Satyananda: The tiger gorges itself on its prey and then regurgitates the remnants of the food from the stomach three to four hours later. There is a good reason for this. The food which is most difficult to digest stays in the stomach longest. The most nutritious and easily digestible food quickly passes through the stomach into the intestines. The remainder contains far less nutrition and its elimination requires a great deal of energy and activity by the digestive organs. The expenditure of the body is probably far greater than the gain. The tiger, therefore, vomits this unrequired portion and avoids overworking the intestines.

The ancient yogis took heed of this sensible habit of the tiger and used it for their own benefit. They took their food in the normal way and three hours later expelled the remaining undigestible or difficult to digest portion. This saved them many intestinal ailments and discomforts and allowed the energy in the body to be directed towards more useful purposes. Vyaghra kriya was also practised most effectively by the later emperors of the Roman Empire, who used it to avoid indigestion after their famous feasts.

Why should vyaghra kriya be performed?

Swami Satyananda: Vyaghra kriya prevents burdening the intestines with undigestible food. However, it has another more obvious use. If bad, rotten, rich or bulky food is eaten the stomach often spontaneously vomits. It is a natural process of the body. This is the last resort of the body for it usually tries to digest the food that has been dumped in the stomach, leading to many hours of heaviness and discomfort. The easiest way to prevent this is to vomit as soon as possible, which sounds a little distasteful but takes only a minute or so and prevents much discomfort. The modern day remedy for indigestion or eating too much rich food is to swallow a tablet. Yet the natural and least harmful way is to vomit. Therefore, vyaghra kriya is recommended to those who want to bring their digestive system quickly back into shape.

In cases of hypoacidity vyaghra dhauti is effective. Hypoacidity causes chronic dyspepsia or indigestion. Due to lack of acidity, the food is not properly digested. When this type of indigestion occurs, three hours after taking food all the remaining contents should be vomited out, leaving the stomach clean.

How is vyaghra kriya performed?

Swami Niranjanananda: If food remains undigested three hours after a meal, at least six glasses of salty lukewarm water are drunk. One then looks up for a few moments before expelling the water. This technique is sometimes called *anna vaman dhauti*, expelling food. Vyaghra kriya is described in *Gheranda Samhita* (1:38–39):

> *Bhojanaante pibedvaari chaakantham pooritam sudheeh.*
> *Urdhvaa drishtim kshanam kritvaa tajjalam vamayetpunah*
>
> *Nityamabhyaasayogena kaphapittam nivaarayet.*
>
> After a meal the practitioner should drink water up to the throat and, after looking upwards for a moment, expel the water by vomiting. (38)
>
> Kapha and pitta disorders are removed. (39)

When should vyaghra kriya be practised?

Swami Niranjanananda: The only purpose of vyaghra kriya is to expel undigested food. It should be done only when necessary. According to yoga, food should pass through the stomach within three hours of eating. If this has not happened, the food is regarded as indigestible and should be thrown out by expulsion. If the food is rotten or the stomach is gorged beyond capacity, the practice can be done earlier. Animals such as lions, tigers and dogs are known to gorge themselves and regurgitate whatever is indigestible.

Vyaghra kriya is only recommended for practice once a week in special circumstances. Twenty-five to thirty minutes after the practice, some light liquid food such as milk or thin *kheer*, rice pudding made with milk, should be eaten.

What precautions should be taken when practising vyaghra kriya?

Swami Niranjanananda: Once food enters the stomach, the sphincter between the stomach and oesophagus is automatically closed and all the energies of the body are focused on moving the food down into the intestines and digesting it. Yogis consider digestion as a function of the downward moving apana vayu, along with the expulsion of waste. Therefore, when food is moved in the opposite direction, as in vyaghra kriya, it must be done under competent guidance, otherwise it can be harmful. Sometimes even healthy people may feel a little pressure in the chest or experience a feeling of burning or acidity.

GAJA KARANI: ELEPHANT ACTION

How can the stomach be cleaned?

Swami Sivananda: Drink a large quantity of water and shake the abdomen. Contract the stomach and vomit the water. This exercise goes by the name *kunjara kriya*. This is a purificatory exercise.

What is gaja karani?

Swami Satyananda: *Gaja karani*, also known as *kunjara kriya*, is an advanced variation of kunjal. Both the words *kunjara* and *gaja* mean 'elephant'. The word *kriya*, means 'practice' or 'action'. Therefore, in English this technique is called the elephant action. It is so-called as it imitates the ability of an elephant to suck in water and expel it at will, although an elephant expels water from the trunk, not from the stomach.

In gaja karani one drinks water and regurgitates it by contracting the upper abdomen while simultaneously inhaling, rather than by rubbing the back of the tongue. It is more difficult than kunjal and does not give any worthwhile advantages over the simpler method.

Gaja karani is described in *Hatha Yoga Pradipika* (2:38):

> *Udaragatapadaarthamudvamanti pavanamapaanamudeerya kanthanaale.*
> *Kramaparichayavashyanaadichakraa gajakaraneeti nigadyate hathajnaih.*
>
> Vomiting the things in the stomach by moving the apana into the throat is called gaja karani by those who have attained knowledge of hatha yoga. Becoming accustomed to this technique, brings about control of the nadis and chakras.

The verse describes a variation of the practice, as it specifies, "vomiting the things in the stomach", indicating that it is practised after eating. It is important that this variation is done three to four hours after eating, so that assimilation of food can take place and then what is difficult to digest is removed before further energy is spent on digestion. This decreases the amount of excrement produced and reduces the workload of the intestines and excretory organs, thereby preventing an overflow of energy in the lower centres. Of course, this practice should not be done after every meal but only as directed by the guru, otherwise it may weaken the digestive system.

How does gaja karani affect the pranic body?

Swami Satyananda: Gaja karani strengthens the solar plexus, the nerve centre which is connected with manipura chakra. Many texts state that all the nadis emanate from the navel region or the 'navel wheel'. The regurgitating reflex pulls the prana up from mooladhara chakra to the throat and stimulates vishuddhi chakra. This upward movement activates all the chakras within the vertebral column and the surrounding nadis. Nerve impulses rush up from the base of the spine to the medulla oblongata and ajna chakra.

VASTRA DHAUTI: CLEANSING WITH CLOTH

What is vastra dhauti?

Swami Satyananda: The word *vastra* means 'cloth' and *dhauti* means 'cleansing' or 'washing'. Therefore, *vastra dhauti* is a technique for cleaning the throat, oesophagus and stomach with a length of cloth dipped in saline water. It is also known by various other names. These include: *vas dhauti*, washing with a cloth, *dhauti kriya*, cleansing technique and *dhauti karma*, cleaning technique.

It is a useful method for removing excess acid or mucus from the stomach. In the past a kind of spongy root was used instead of a cloth. Vastra dhauti is described in *Hatha Yoga Pradipika* (2:24):

> *Chaturangulavistaaram hastapanchadashaayatam.*
> *Guroopadishtamaargena siktam vastram shanairgraset.*
> *Punah pratyaaharechchaitaduditam dhauti karma tat.*
>
> A strip of wet cloth, four angulas wide (seven to eight centimetres) and fifteen handspans (one and a half metres) in length is slowly swallowed and then taken out, as instructed by the guru. This is known as dhauti.

If one's legs are reasonably flexible, a squatting position is ideal when peforming this practice. Otherwise one may sit on a low stool or chair. Vastra dhauti must only be practised under expert guidance and in full accordance with the instructions given. Those who practise varisara dhauti need not do vastra dhauti.

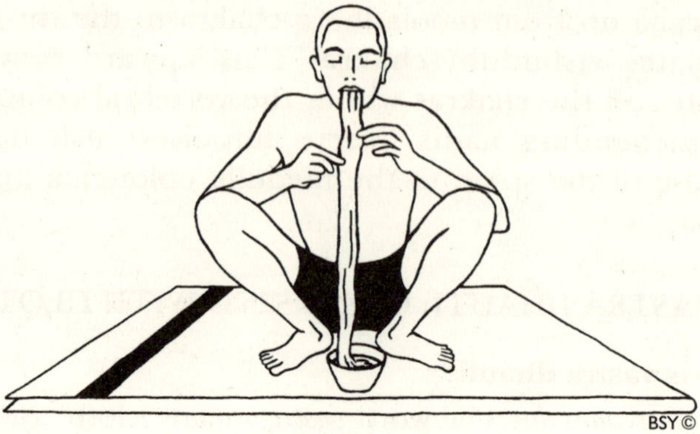

Vastra Dhauti

What type of cloth is used for vastra dhauti?

Swami Satyananda: The cloth should be of finely woven cotton which is unused and perfectly clean. Synthetic material should definitely not be used and the cloth should not be dyed. White muslin is ideal. The cloth must also be trimmed neatly so that no loose threads fray on the sides.

The same cloth can be used again and again. After the practice, thoroughly wash the cloth, dry it and store it in a safe, clean place.

How is the cloth prepared for vastra dhauti?

Swami Niranjanananda: Care must be taken with all the preparations and stages of the practice. Ensure that enough time is available for the practice to be performed without any disturbance. To learn vastra dhauti, the guidance of an experienced teacher is essential.

The cloth used for the practice of this dhauti kriya should be four fingers wide, i.e. about eight to ten centimetres, and at least six metres in length. It should be cotton and very thin and soft, not at all rough. Beginners should start with a roll just two and a half centimetres wide and three metres long. When the practice can be done easily, the length and width of the cloth can be increased.

When cutting the cloth to the required size, ensure that all the loose fibres along the edges are removed properly so they do not get stuck inside the stomach. It is possible to buy a sterile, lightweight cotton bandage from a chemist for the purpose, but it should be checked carefully for loose threads.

The cloth must be prepared with maximum care. After cutting and removing any loose fibres, the cloth is washed and boiled in water, then soaked in lukewarm water so that it becomes even softer. Some people soak the roll either in milk or milk mixed with sugar. If this method makes the practice easier, it can be used for a few days to help prepare the mind, otherwise plain hot water is best. In *Gheranda Samhita* (1:40) it is written:

> *Chaturangula vistaaram sookshmavastram shanairgraset;*
> *Punah pratyaaharedetatprochyate dhautikarmakam.*
>
> A roll of fine cotton cloth four fingers wide should be gradually swallowed and then taken out slowly.

Is nauli kriya used during the practice of vastra dhauti?
Swami Niranjanananda: Stage two of vastra dhauti involves nauli kriya. After swallowing the cloth, nauli is performed, keeping the cloth inside. Initially this abdominal churning should only be practised for one minute. Even an experienced practitioner should not practise nauli for more than five minutes. The cloth should not be kept inside the abdomen any longer as it could slip down into the intestines. The abdomen is rotated or churned so that the cloth reaches all parts of the stomach and collects *kapha* and *pitta*, mucus and excess digestive juices. After that, the cloth is slowly pulled out.

When and how often should vastra dhauti be performed?
Swami Niranjanananda: According to the rules of yoga this practice should not be done more than once a week. It is not to be done daily. It should be practised when the stomach is completely empty. An appropriate time is before breakfast.

What are the health benefits of vastra dhauti?

Swami Satyananda: The cloth thoroughly scrubs the stomach walls. It stimulates the digestive juices and peristalsis, and invigorates the entire body. It is useful in treating acidity, indigestion, bronchitis and asthma.

For maximum benefit, kunjal kriya and jala neti should be performed after completing vastra dhauti. Vastra dhauti scrapes the impurities from the walls, while kunjal expels them from the body. Jala neti tones up the nasal system.

What is the purpose of practising vastra dhauti?

Swami Niranjanananda: Vastra dhauti is a method of cleaning the throat, oesophagus and stomach with a length of cloth. Even though the practice is difficult, it remains prevalent due to its many benefits. Sage Gheranda says that this technique cures kapha and pitta disorders and is also useful for kidney problems, leprosy and skin infections. It is especially effective for those who suffer from asthma. In *Gheranda Samhita* (1:41) it is written:

> *Gulma jvarapleehaakushthakaphapittam vinashyati;*
> *Aarogyam balapushtishcha bhavettasya dine dine.*
>
> The practice of vastra dhauti rectifies skin problems, fever, enlarged spleen, leprosy and kapha (phlegm) and pitta (bile) disorders. It keeps the body free of disease, increases stamina and cheerfulness, and promotes healthy growth.

Vastra dhauti is the only example of dhauti described in Yogi Swatmarama's *Hatha Yoga Pradipika*, which perhaps shows the usefulness of the practice.

Many people begin yoga due to interest in improving their health through its cleansing practices. For both Yogi Swatmarama and Sage Gheranda, however, their real aim in teaching these practices is as part of yoga sadhana, preparing the practitioner for pranayama and higher practices.

Why is vastra dhauti particularly recommended for the relief of asthma?

Swami Niranjanananda: The practice of vastra dhauti affects the entire body and is a time-tested cure for people who suffer from kapha disorders or excess phlegm, such as asthmatics. Vastra dhauti is essential for the prevention and cure of asthma.

It may be wondered why this practice is helpful, given that asthma is a disorder of the respiratory system, and vastra dhauti directly affects the digestive system. The answer lies in the fact that nerves and nadis link the digestive system with the lungs and brain. It should be remembered that the nervous system, including the brain, plays an important role in asthma. It is not just the respiratory system or the lungs that are affected.

How often should vastra dhauti be practised for the relief of asthma?

Swami Satyananda: Those who suffer from asthma can practise vastra dhauti daily for two weeks during times of acute attacks. After this, once a week is sufficient. It is simple but effective for both the prevention and cure of asthma. Many asthmatics gain relief using this practice.

What precautions should be taken when practising vastra dhauti?

Swami Niranjanananda: The cloth should always be kept in close contact with the tongue. If it is in contact with the palate, it obstructs respiration, triggers a cough reflex and the cloth comes out.

The second precaution is that the cloth, lubricated with saliva, should be passed down the throat bit by bit. It is helpful to drink a little water in between. Initially the cloth may keep coming out and it may take some practice before being able to swallow it. With courage and patience the student must keep trying to swallow the cloth, and eventually the technique will be mastered

After practising for a few days or weeks the cloth will start sliding down the oesophagus quite quickly. Always ensure that at least 30 cm of cloth remains outside and keep a firm hold of it.

A seasoned practitioner of vastra dhauti can swallow a length of cloth twelve arms in length in just five minutes. Once swallowed, the cloth should not remain in the stomach for more than five minutes. On completion, it must be slowly pulled out.

What are the contra-indications for the practice of vastra dhauti?

Swami Niranjanananda: Vastra dhauti practice should not be performed by people suffering from hypertension, heart disease, stroke, peptic ulcer, gastritis, during illness or when the body is in a weakened state. It should not be practised until six months after surgery, or during pregnancy.

When should vastra dhauti be practised rather than kunjal?

Swami Niranjanananda: Vastra dhauti is a stronger practice than kunjal and can sometimes improve conditions that are beyond the scope of kunjal. However, it is also more difficult to perform. In the beginning this practice must be done under the guidance of a competent teacher.

When the cloth comes out, it is no longer thin, but quite thick, as it brings kapha or mucus with it. This does not always happen in kunjal. When the cloth is pulled out, it looks as if it is completely drenched in ghee, and feels slippery from top to bottom. The cloth wipes the walls of the stomach thoroughly, which enables digestive juices to be efficiently secreted.

How long does it take to master vastra dhauti?

Swami Satyananda: Vastra dhauti cannot be mastered on the first day. It may take a few days or even a few weeks before the whole length of cloth can be swallowed. It is strange but true that the less one tries the easier it becomes; the more one relaxes the more easily the cloth goes down the throat. If one forgets that the cloth is a piece of cloth and merely swallows, the cloth will automatically drop into the stomach. There is no hurry, it is best to take one's time.

The beginner should practise daily for about ten minutes whether the cloth can be swallowed or not. After a few days one becomes used to the cloth entering the throat. When the mind accepts the idea, it is but a short step to mastering the technique.

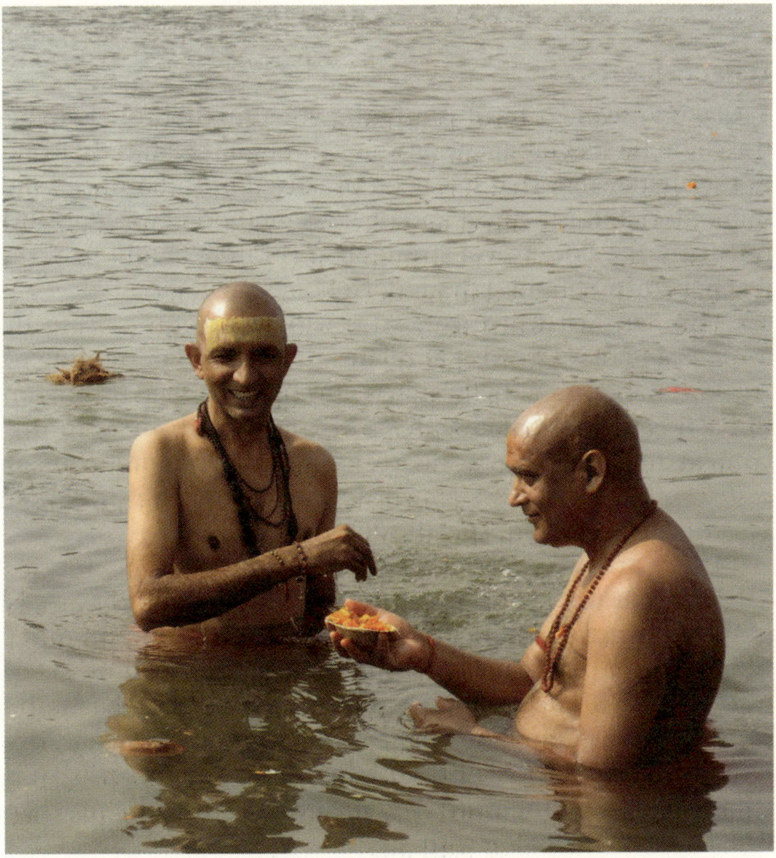

8

Basti: Yogic Enema

WHAT IS BASTI?

What is basti?

Swami Satyananda: Basti is a hatha yoga method of cleaning the colon by sucking in air or water through the anus. It is one of the shatkarmas that has been practised in India since time immemorial. It is a direct and obvious method of washing and purifying the bowels, yet strangely it is rarely taught by yoga teachers or mentioned in modern books on yoga.

The Sanskrit word *basti*, also widely written as *vasti* or *wasti*, is a general word that relates to anything pertaining to the lower abdomen, belly, pelvis and bladder. The technique of basti is widely called *basti karma*. The word *karma* in this context means 'process' or 'technique'. Therefore, *basti* or *basti karma* is a process concerned with cleaning the lower part of the abdomen, specifically the colon.

There are two types of basti, sthala and jala:

1. *Sthala basti*: The word *sthala* means 'ground'. Sthala basti is a practice where one stands on dry ground; in other words, it is a practice where one sucks air, instead of water, into the anus. The technique is also called sushka basti, the word *sushka* meaning 'dry'. Therefore, *sushka basti* means 'dry basti' or more exactly 'air basti'. Another name for air basti is vata basti, where the word *vata* means 'air'. It is the practice which cleans the colon with air.

2. *Jala basti*: The word *jala* means 'water', therefore jala basti is the practice where one sucks water into the anus. It is also called vari basti, *vari* meaning 'water'. Therefore, vari basti is the process of cleaning the colon with water. In *Gheranda Samhita* (1:45) it is written:

Jala vastih shushkavastirvastee cha dvividhau smritau;
Jala vastim jale kuryaachchhushkavastim sadaa kshitau.

The practice of basti is of two types: water (jala) basti and dry (sthala) basti. Jala basti is done in water. Dry basti is done on land, in a dry place.

Why is basti known as a yogic enema?

Swami Niranjanananda: Basti is a simple practice for washing and purifying the intestines. It is like a yogic enema, as air or water is sucked in through the anus in order to clean the large intestine.

The water does not enter the small intestine, but remains in the large intestine. After some time the water is expelled, just as in a regular enema. The only difference is that in an enema a tube is used. Basti is more natural and more appropriate. In *Hatharatnavali* (1:41–44), the two types of basti are described:

Vastistu dvividhaa proktaa jalavaayu prabhedatah.
Chakrim kritvaa yathaashaktyaa vastinchaiva tu kaarayet.

Vaayumaakunchya jathare gudanaale visarjayet
Vaayuvastiriyam proktaa jalavasti matho bruve.

Atha jalavastih
Naabhidadhne jale sthitvaa paayunaale sthitaangulih.
Chakrimaargena jatharam paayunaalena poorayet.

Vichitrakaraneem kritvaa nirbheeto rechayejjalam.
Yaavadbalam pooryaiva kshanam sthitvaa virechayent.

Basti is said to be of two types: water and air. After doing chakrikarma according to the best of one's effort, one should practise basti. (41)

After collecting air in the stomach, release it through the lower passage (anus). Vayu basti is explained; Now I will speak about jala basti. (42)

Now jala basti: Standing in water up to the navel region, put the finger in the passage of the anus. Through the chakri process, the stomach should be filled with water through the anus. (43)

Then, after doing vichitra karani, one should draw out the water without fear. Draw the water according to your strength, wait for some moments then expel it. (44)

How does jala basti work?
Swami Niranjanananda: To practise jala basti, the sphincter muscles are carefully expanded to their maximum to allow the inward flow of water. It is likely that only a little water will go inside the first time basti is practised. But as control over the muscles increases, with greater contraction and expansion taking place, more water will enter the body and then come out, making a rumbling sound. Initially, waste material sticking to the walls of the rectum (the final, almost straight part of the large intestine) is expelled. Next, the water brings out dried, hardened waste that has collected inside, thus cleansing the large intestine.

What is the difference between jala basti and an enema?
Swami Niranjanananda: Many people unknowingly resort to a variation of jala basti. They take an enema by inserting the spout of a tube into the anus and keep the water level high in the tube so that the pressure of the water is felt inside. When the spout is removed, both water and waste matter come out.

The difference is that in jala basti one is not inserting a spout, but rather developing muscular control to bring water into the body. There is also the invigorating and rejuvenating effect of standing in running water during the more natural basti technique.

TECHNIQUES

What is the general method for practising basti?

Swami Satyananda: The method is exactly the same for both jala and sthala basti. The only difference is that jala basti is practised in water and sthala basti in air. The full practice can be summarized as follows:

Stage 1: initial suction and evacuation of air or water.

Stage 2: progressive suction; in this stage a greater amount of water or air is drawn into the colon in order to bring about the best possible wash.

Stage 3: rotational nauli; the technique of rotational nauli (stage 2 of nauli) should be integrated with basti. If one cannot do rotational nauli, either agnisar kriya, uddiyana bandha, bhastrika pranayama or madhyama nauli can be performed. In these alternative practices the abdominal muscles should be rhythmically contracted and relaxed. Rotational nauli is the preferred practice.

Stage 4: evacuate the water or air and stool mixture into a toilet. Then do *mayurasana*, peacock pose, or *hamsasana*, swan pose. These two asanas exert pressure on the colon, ensuring full evacuation and stimulating intestinal peristalsis. One then goes to the toilet again to empty the bowels.

If the water is dirty, the whole process, stages one to four, can be repeated. This is the complete practice of basti, for both jala and sthala.

What practices prepare one for basti?

Swami Satyananda: In order to perform basti one must develop control over the abdominal muscles by practising yogic techniques such as bhastrika pranayama, uddiyana bandha and asanas in general.

Before attempting basti, madhyama nauli should be mastered. This is necessary in order to suck water or air into the colon.

How difficult is it to learn jala basti?

Swami Niranjanananda: This practice is highly beneficial, and it is not difficult. The technique is described in *Gheranda Samhita* (1:46):

> *Naabhimagnajale paayunyastanaalotkataasanah;*
> *Aakunchanam prasaaram cha jala vastim samaacharet.*
>
> Sitting in water up to the navel, adopt utkatasana, then contract and expand the anal region. This is jala basti.

As *utkatasana* is a half standing and half squatting position, the anus can be more easily and fully contracted and expanded in coordination with the breath. Jala basti should be practised without stress, and undue force should never be applied, although the sphincter muscles should fully open the anus.

Why should basti be practised in a flowing river?

Swami Niranjanananda: In ayurveda, as well as in yoga, water is used in abundance for purifying and curing the body. When the authors of the hatha yoga texts were teaching many centuries ago, there were abundant sources of pure water in rivers and streams and this practice was performed in a natural and uplifting setting. The problem is that today a suitable environment for the practice cannot be found and so the modern alternative of health salons and the essentially passive use of enemas has been developed as a substitute.

In one sense jala basti is just a practice of *ashwini mudra*: contraction and expansion of the anus. It is, however, synchronized with the breath while standing in deep water up to the navel. Pure water has many natural therapeutic qualities. Flowing water like that of a pure river is best, as the waste product which comes out during the practice is immediately washed away by the flowing water. The pressure exerted by flowing water also influences the practice. Basti must not be practised in a polluted river.

For optimal practice one should stand in deep, fresh flowing water up to the navel and adopt utkatasana. Unfortunately it is now extremely difficult to find a suitable water supply free from pollution. If such a place is found, it should be protected rather than polluting it with one's own bodily wastes. Therefore, the practice of basti must be adapted by practising in a bath or tub, or by using a tube to suck the water up from a container.

How should one prepare the water for jala basti?

Swami Satyananda: For water basti one has to sit or stand in a bath of water unless a tube is used. The water level should be such that it is just above the level of the anus. The depth of water required will depend on the sitting position. For example, if sitting in paschimottanasana five to ten centimetres is sufficient whereas if one is standing in utkatasana, the water needs to be much deeper.

The water should be neither excessively cold nor hot. If there is sufficient time one can use warm water first (body temperature is ideal) to loosen hard encrusted stool from the walls of the colon, then cooler water (not freezing); to tone up the nerves of the colon and anus, and stimulate blood circulation. This is useful for those who suffer from piles or constipation.

Is abdominal breathing used to help draw water inside during basti?

Swami Niranjanananda: The abdomen should not be moved with the breath; only the anus is contracted and expanded. On inhalation the anus is pulled inside and on exhalation the anus is totally relaxed – contraction and expansion.

How long is water retained inside during jala basti?

Swami Satyananda: If there is time the water can be retained inside the colon for five or ten minutes before practising nauli. Retaining the water further helps to remove stool that has become encrusted on the intestinal walls.

What is involved in the practice of sthala, or dry basti?

Swami Niranjanananda: For the practice of sthala basti, the anus is contracted and expanded by practising ashwini mudra while sitting on the ground. This is described in *Gheranda Samhita* (1:48):

> *Paschimottaanato vastim chaalayitvaa shanaih shanaih;*
> *Ashvineemudrayaa paayumaakunchayetprasaarayet.*
>
> Sitting in paschimottanasana, practise basti in the lower portion, contracting and expanding the anus by means of ashwini mudra.

The asana mentioned here is *paschimottanasana*, the back stretching pose, but it is adjusted slightly to *utthanpadasana*, the stretched leg pose, which can be called simple paschimottanasana. In this position *ashwini mudra*, contraction and expansion of the anus, is performed, to suck air inside the body.

While inhaling, the anus is pulled in and up and the sphincter muscles are contracted. On exhalation the anus is expanded. During inhalation the chest is expanded and the diaphragm consciously pulled upwards. It is relaxed on exhalation. This helps pull air into the rectum.

How can one prepare the body for sthala basti?

Swami Niranjanananda: Hatha yoga texts suggest that a tube can be used if there is initial difficulty sucking in air. Ghee is applied to a rubber tube which is then gently inserted into the anus. The anal muscles are expanded with the help of the fingers, so that the rubber tube can be inserted easily and the possibility of injury is ruled out. There should be no tension and the anal muscles should be allowed to expand in a natural way. The tube must not be inserted too deeply in case it is sucked in completely. Do not practise ashwini mudra, instead focus on the breath.

During inhalation, as the chest expands the abdominal muscles are pulled in and up. This creates a negative pressure, a type of vacuum, inside the abdomen. When this negative pressure is created, air is sucked upwards automatically via the tube. During exhalation, push the diaphragm down, without straining, so that pressure is created within the abdomen and air is expelled through the tube.

Once experience has been gained with the help of the tube, the practitioner will have a feeling for which type of pressure needs to be created inside and with which type of pressure the air is to be expelled. Once the practice has been learned, stop using the tube. It is essential that ashwini mudra is not performed when using a tube to avoid the possibility of the tube being sucked inside.

Which way of practising basti is preferable?

Swami Satyananda: Water basti is a better practice than air basti since it thoroughly scrubs the intestinal walls. Air basti does not clean the walls of the bowels; rather it helps to stimulate intestinal peristalsis in order to remove accumulated stool. Both are useful for constipation. Air basti has the advantage that it can be practised anywhere, without preparation.

What should one do if basti cannot be practised?

Swami Satyananda: If it is not possible to practise either jala or sthala basti, moola shodhana is advised. A douche may also be inserted into the rectum or an enema used. An enema cleans the colon, but basti allows the heat of the abdomen to be eliminated and absorbed by the water that one is standing in. In India, basti is traditionally practised in a flowing river.

GUIDELINES FOR PRACTICE

Is basti suitable for everyone?

Swami Niranjanananda: Basti is not suitable for everyone. It is contra-indicated for high blood pressure, hernia and any serious disorder related to digestion, such as inflammatory bowel disease or bowel cancer. Basti is beneficial for some common diseases, including constipation, diarrhoea and irritable bowel syndrome. Anyone suffering from diseases of the abdomen should seek guidance from an expert.

Although it is easy to describe, basti must only be practised under the guidance of a competent and qualified teacher.

When and how often should basti be practised?

Swami Niranjanananda: Both jala and sthala basti can be practised at any time of day, but ideally they are performed in the morning before breakfast. If there is sufficient time, the practice should be continued until clean water, rather than waste product, starts coming out.

Basti should be undertaken only when required. If one suffers from constipation, once a week is sufficient for general cleansing. Basti should not become a daily habit. Some waste product should remain in the large intestines as certain bacteria are required for maintaining the general health of the body. Excessive practice of basti interferes with the growth of bacteria, irritates the lining of the large intestine and may harm the muscles of the anus and large intestine.

Why is basti only practised during warm weather?

Swami Niranjanananda: Jala basti removes physical heat. The water absorbs the internal body heat, so that when it comes gushing out, body heat is lost. This discharge of physical heat cannot be restored immediately during cold weather.

Many people have found that if basti is practised during cloudy, windy or stormy weather, when the external temperature is unstable, constipation occurs due to the inability of the body to recuperate from the loss of body heat. Therefore, it is recommended that the practice of basti only be done when the weather is warm or hot.

Can jala basti be practised with the use of a tube?

Swami Satyananda: One traditional method of doing basti is to insert a thin bamboo tube into the anus. This allows air or water to be sucked easily into the colon via the anus. The boon of modern technology means that a thin plastic tube can be used. In fact plastic is preferable to bamboo since it is smoother and more flexible. Bamboo could be a little harsh on the sphincter muscles of the anus. In *Hatha Yoga Pradipika* (2:26) jala basti is described with the use of a tube:

> *Naabhidaghnajale paayau nyastanaalotkataasanah.*
> *Aadhaaraakunchanam kuryaatkshaalanam bastikarma tat.*
>
> Sitting in utkatasana, navel deep in water, insert a tube into the anus and contract the anus. This cleansing with water is called basti karma.

The use of a tube is a good method if one takes care. However, it is much safer and much easier to merely open the anal sphincters with the fingers.

The use of a tube for jala basti has one big advantage: water can be sucked up into the colon from a container. This means basti can be practised without standing in a river or a deep bath.

Why is basti preferable to an enema?

Swami Satyananda: The most common method of using an enema is gravity feed. Water or whatever is being used as the enema is kept in a container above the level of the anus. A thin tube feeds the water from the container directly into the anus. The water flows directly into the colon under the force of gravity, no effort is necessary.

The gravity feed method is similar to basti and is certainly much easier. Basti requires some degree of muscular control. If a person has severe constipation and cannot do basti, they should adopt the gravity feed method. However, mastering basti is recommended since it has the following advantages:

- It develops strength and control of the abdominal muscles, which is necessary in order to suck the air or water into the bowels. This in itself helps to improve the efficiency and health of the abdominal organs.

- It simultaneously massages the inner organs and tones up the nerves.
- It requires little or no equipment.

If one can do basti, with or without a tube, it is preferable to a gravity feed enema.

What postures can be used for practising basti?

Swami Satyananda: The following asanas can be used while doing basti. Choose whichever asana is suitable:

Utkatasana, unyielding pose: this is the asana in which one practises nauli and is the traditional method recommended by *Gheranda Samhita* and *Hatha Yoga Pradipika*. It can be used for jala and sthala basti, but if it is used for jala basti, the water has to be deep.

Kagasana, crow pose: this is the squatting pose. It is an ideal position for sucking in both air and water. Less than thirty centimetres of water is required.

Paschimottanasana, back stretching pose. A simplified version of the full form of this asana can be used for basti. One should sit on the ground for air basti or in water for jala basti. It does not matter if the head cannot touch the knees. The important thing is that the deepest possible exhalation is attained; this is mainly achieved by contracting the abdominal muscles. The purpose of leaning forwards in paschimottanasana is only to achieve greater expulsion of air from the lungs. This sitting position has two main advantages: it can be practised in shallow water, even less than eight centimetres, and it can be easily and comfortably practised by almost everyone.

How does one suck water or air into the anus?

Swami Satyananda: The method of sucking water or air into the anus is difficult to describe. One must try it in order to understand it. After exhaling fully, the breath is held out and the anal sphincter is gently opened with the fingers.

Madhyama nauli is then practised whilst trying to expand and pull up the abdomen. This process creates a vacuum and sucks in water or air. As water is drawn in, the anal muscles are gently manipulated so that there is free flow through the anus.

Some people can do this technique the first time; others require a lot of practice. It is easy when one knows how.

How often should basti be practised if stool is not passed daily?

Swami Satyananda: Daily use of basti or any other form of enema is absolutely not necessary. Many people think that their colon has to be perfectly clean. They develop a neurosis if they do not go to the toilet every morning. For this reason they resort to the daily use of an enema or laxative. Try to avoid this drastic measure and do not worry if stool is not passed every day.

What are the dietary guidelines following basti?

Swami Niranjanananda: In *Hatharatnavali* (1:45) it says food should not be eaten for three *ghatis*, about one and a quarter hours, after the practice of basti:

> *Ghatitrayam na bhoktavyam vastimabhyasyato dhruvam.*
> *Nivaatabhoomau santishthedvashee hitamitaashanah.*
>
> After practising basti one should not take a meal for three ghatis (seventy-two minutes). He should sit peacefully on the ground and take controlled, pleasurable and moderate food.

BENEFITS

What are the health benefits of practising jala basti?

Swami Sivananda: Jala basti cures urinary disorders, dyspepsia, disorders of digestion, diseases of the bowels, and diseases arising from an excess of wind, bile and phlegm. This kriya should be done in the morning when the stomach is empty.

What are the general benefits of intestinal cleansing with basti?

Swami Satyananda: Basti is the best method for cleansing the bowels and is a great help in reducing the occurrence of various types of disease as well as improving general health. It is generally believed that a large number of ailments originate in the colon, especially from impurities and malfunction. Actually most ailments arise in the mind, but certainly a congested colon or excessive toxins in the bowels can help to initiate ailments. Basti completely washes the bowel and removes excess bacteria, old stool, threadworms and heat from the lower intestines.

Basti stimulates the nerves of the colon as well as the nerves connecting other parts and organs of the digestive system. It also improves muscle tone and blood supply. Old stool and gas are removed and the blood is purified. Once basti has been practised and mastered it can be used occasionally for general health or to treat specific ailments such as constipation.

Basti cures digestive disorders and is particularly useful for removing constipation, stimulating sluggish digestion, controlling nervous diarrhoea and strengthening the solar plexus.

Most importantly, it pushes apana vayu upward. When the apana rises it can be felt in the navel region and as a great pressure on the stomach. In *Hatha Yoga Pradipka* (2:27–28) it is written:

> *Gulmapleehodaram chaapi vaatapittakaphodbhavaah.*
> *Bastikarmaprabhaavena ksheeyante sakalaamayaah.*
>
> *Dhaatvindriyaantahkaranaprasaadam daghaachcha kaantim dahanapradeeptim.*
> *Asheshadoshopachayam nihanyaadabhyasyamaanam jala-bastikarma.*
>
> Enlargement of the glands and spleen, and all diseases arising from excess wind, bile and mucus are eliminated from the body through the practice of basti. (27)

By practising jala basti the appetite increases, the body glows, excess doshas are destroyed and the dhatu, senses and mind are purified. (28)

What is the best method for cleansing the large intestine?

Swami Niranjanananda: Basti is the best technique for cleansing the large intestine. In *Gheranda Samhita* (1:49) it is written:

> *Evamabhyaasayogena koshthadosho na vidyate;*
> *Vivarddhayejjatharaagnimaamavaatam vinaashayet.*
>
> It removes diseases of the stomach and bowels and enhances the digestive fire.

Evamabhyaasayogena koshthadosho na vidyate, by this practice constipation is prevented in a yogi's body. Disorders of the stomach and intestines do not occur. *Vivarddhayejjatharaagnimaamavaatam vinaashayet*, diseases which manifest due to lack of digestive fire, like flatulence, indigestion, constipation, and pitta and kapha imbalances, are eradicated.

Basti enhances the energy and helps develop control over the abdominal muscles. To suck up water or air requires muscular control. There is a clear improvement in the health and capacity of the abdominal organs with this practice alone. Blood circulation takes place efficiently so that the exchange of oxygen and waste is optimized, and the blood is purified. The internal organs are massaged, making the nadis healthy.

What are the physical and pranic benefits of basti?

Swami Niranjanananda: In *Gheranda Samhita* (1:47), the benefits of basti are described:

> *Prameham cha udaavartam krooravaayum nivaarayet;*
> *Bhavetsvachchhandadehashcha kaamadevasamo bhavet.*
>
> This practice removes wind disorders, urinary and digestive problems, and makes the body beautiful like that of Kamadeva, the god of love.

Disorders like *prameha*, intestinal problems, haemorrhoids and unhealthy wind, here termed *kroora vayu*, are removed and the physical body is purified. A light and radiant body like that of Kamadeva, the god of love, or Cupid, is attained when toxic waste is removed from the body. Good health definitely increases the glow and lustre of the body.

Many nadis in the body terminate near the anus. When sensations take place in those nadis, the entire nervous system is activated, and increased sensitivity and energy are experienced. Basti stimulates the pranic energy and one feels active and dynamic afterwards.

Yogis have experienced a drop in body temperature when water is sucked into the anus, as the body's internal heat is reduced. This reduces boils, which often form due to excessive internal heat. Some skin diseases, like the forms of 'dry' dermatitis in which the skin cracks, and blood and pus flow, are cured. Note that this does not include 'wet' skin conditions in which there is oozing of watery fluid.

Udaavartam is upward moving wind. Often when the bowels are full of wind, it cannot be expelled despite considerable effort. This wind causes pressure on the right side of the abdomen, especially in the lower part where the appendix is located, causing pain in that area. This disorder is common in small children, and when the abdomen is massaged, the wind is expelled with a rumbling sound through the anus or by belching from the mouth. This wind can also be removed through the practice of jala basti.

Can shankhaprakshalana be practised instead of basti?

Swami Niranjanananda: Given that the practices of dhauti, including shankhaprakshalana, are given as a means of purifying the whole body, it may be asked what is the need for basti? If there is constipation, shankhaprakshalana can be performed and the digestive tract will be cleaned properly from top to bottom. However, shankhaprakshalana should only be practised once every six months, whereas basti may be undertaken regularly to remove constipation and clear the bowels while the problem persists.

What is the best treatment for severe constipation?

Swami Satyananda: If the constipation is serious, basti should be preceded by moola shodhana. This practice will remove hard stool. Water basti can then be used to thoroughly clean the bowels. Basti may also bring some relief from pruritis (itching of the anus).

Is basti useful for the relief of haemorrhoids?

Swami Niranjanananda: People suffering from haemorrhoids should practise jala basti with care. Cold water should be used as it will cause constriction of the blood vessels, which are dilated in haemorrhoids, and bring immediate relief. Many ailments of the anus benefit from basti.

Why is basti practised before fasting?

Swami Niranjanananda: If a fast is planned to purify the body, practising basti before starting the fast will enable maximum purification.

How does basti help one prepare for higher yogic practices?

Swami Satyananda: Jala basti is especially important for those who wish to do the higher practices of yoga.

By practising basti the abdominal functions can be improved. There are many diseases of the abdominal area. An aspirant should aspire to be free of them if he wishes to sit for any length of time in meditation poses. The condition of the stomach influences the thought patterns and can bring about negative sensations and visions. During a deep psychic state of mind, one might see an elephant flying, or himself falling down from the top of a hill. Such experiences are likely to interrupt the meditation.

Sometimes meditation is practised for a long time in padmasana or siddhasana, causing heat in mooladhara or the rectum, even a long time before the kundalini is aroused. This sensation of heat can be felt by touch. It should be reduced, as it can have repercussions in the brain, making the awakening of kundalini dangerous. Before psychic awakening is to take place, therefore, the abdominal condition should be absolutely normal, so that the lower portion of the body is not heated. Therefore, basti karma, the process of abdominal purification, is prescribed.

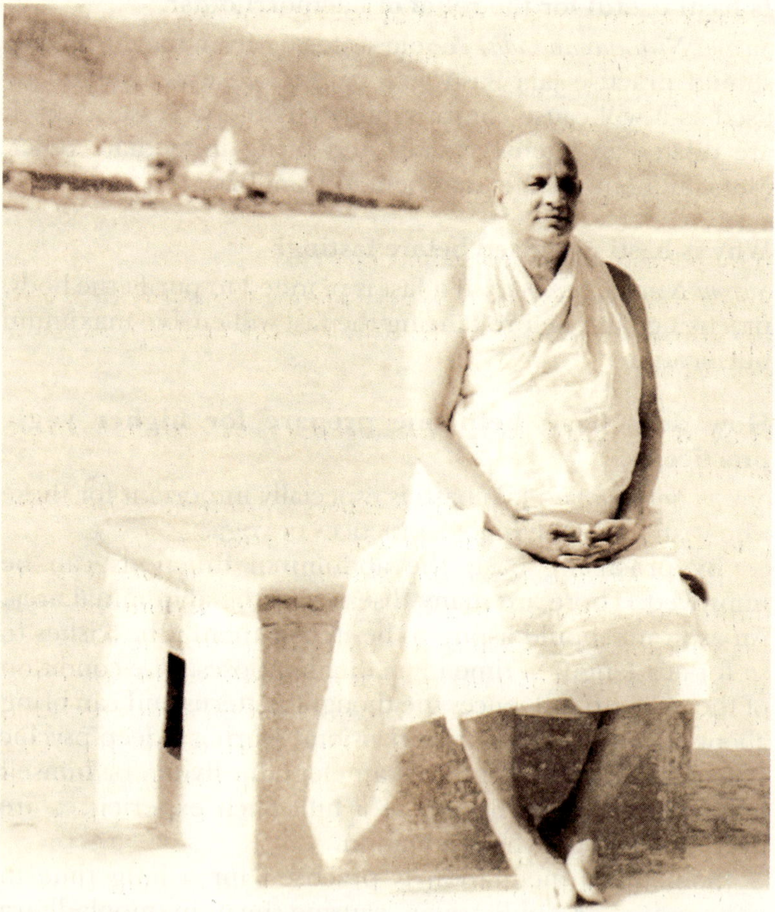

9

Nauli: Abdominal Massage

WHAT IS NAULI?

What is nauli?

Swami Satyananda: Nauli is a yogic technique of massaging the entire abdomen and stomach by contracting and rolling the abdominal muscles. It is a technique in which the rectus abdominis are pressed against the surface of the stomach like the trunk of a bamboo tree. The projected muscles are rotated in a circular movement from left to right, and from right to left for about ten to fifteen minutes. In *Hatharatnavali* (1:32) it is written:

> *Atha baahyaakhyaa naulih*
> *Amandaavartavegena tundham savyaapasavyatah.*
> *Nataamso bhraamayedeshaa naulirgaundaih prashasyate.*
>
> With shoulders bent forward one should rotate the abdomen (muscles) right and left with the speed of a fast rotating whirlpool. This nauli is praised by the accomplished yogis.

What does nauli look like when practised correctly?

Swami Sivananda: When nauli is demonstrated by an advanced yogic student, onlookers are extremely surprised at the movements of the abdominal muscles. It looks as if an engine is working in the abdominal factory.

What is the literal translation of the word 'nauli'?

Swami Satyananda: The Sanskrit word nauli comes from the root word *nala* or *nali*, which means a tubular vessel, vein or nerve of the body, or, a reed or hollow stalk, perhaps of a lotus. The word *nala* is also Sanskrit for the rectus abdominis muscles – in the Monier Williams *Sanskrit-English Dictionary* it is literally defined as the 'navel string'. The rectus abdominis are the two muscles which act as pillars supporting the abdominal organs between the pelvic region and the chest. Thus *nauli* is the technique that is concerned with manipulation of the rectus abdominis muscles.

It is also interesting to note that the Sanskrit word *nau* means 'ship'. When nauli is perfected, the abdominal muscles seem to flow like the rolling waves of the ocean. The muscles create the same wave-like motion produced by a ship gliding through the water.

Nauli is also called *lauliki karma*. The word *lauliki* is derived from the root word *lola* which means 'to move hither and thither', or, 'rolling and agitation'. This is exactly what the technique of lauliki does. It rolls, rotates and agitates the entire abdomen and associated muscles and nerves. The word karma here means 'process or technique'. Thus lauliki karma is the technique of rotating the abdominal muscles and stirring up the inner organs.

What is lauliki?

Swami Niranjanananda: The word *lauliki* is derived from the root *lola*, meaning to roll or agitate, and in this practice the abdomen is rotated and contracted so that all the abdominal organs as well as the muscles and ligaments are stimulated and activated. Another name for this practice is *nauli kriya*. The abdominal muscles are squeezed in, and the muscles on first the left and then the right sides, are strongly constricted. In *Gheranda Samhita* (1:52) lauliki is briefly described:

Amandavegena tundam bhraamayedubhapaarshvayoh;
Sarvarogaannihanteeha dehaanalavivarddhanam.

The abdomen should be rotated swiftly from side to side. This lauliki (nauli) destroys all types of diseases and activates the digestive fire.

Lauliki is a powerful technique which massages and strengthens all the abdominal organs and should be practised by those suffering from indigestion, loss of appetite or intestinal worms. It is also useful for removing excess *vata* or wind. The practice increases the digestive fire. As a result it benefits the entire digestive system and overall health. It is difficult for beginners, but can be mastered with resolve and regular practice.

Are uddiyana bandha, agnisar kriya and nauli kriya related practices?

Swami Niranjanananda: After the intestines have been cleansed and their optimum health guaranteed by the practice of basti, the next shatkarma is nauli, rotation of the stomach muscles. Nauli is a kriya, and kriya is a part of bandha.

Bandhas are postural contractions of the body, such as the chin lock, the stomach lock and the perineal lock. *Kriyas* are moving contractions, both preparatory and advanced

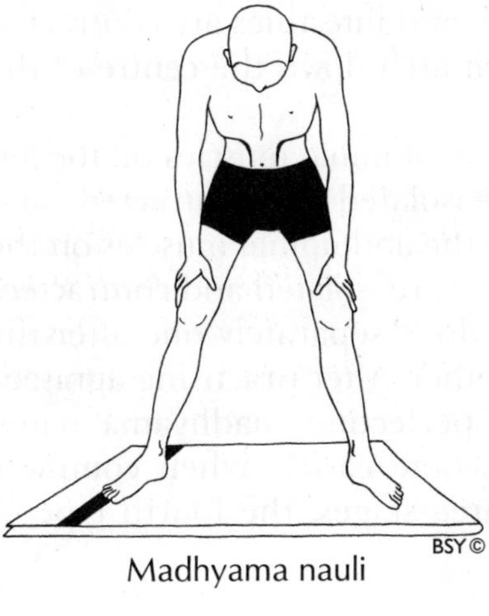

Madhyama nauli

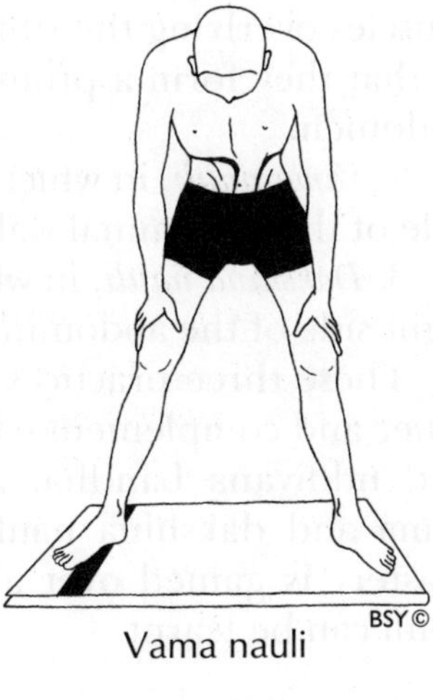

Vama nauli

techniques of bandhas. One example is agnisar kriya. *Agnisar kriya* is a simple practice of emptying the lungs and holding the breath outside while pumping the stomach in and out as many times as possible, then inhaling deeply and relaxing. The rapid contraction of the lower abdominal muscles strengthens the diaphragm and the lower stomach region, and prepares the body for the practice of uddiyana bandha.

Nauli is an advanced version of uddiyana bandha. In nauli the muscles of the abdomen are pulled together at the centre of the lower abdomen and can be seen externally in the form of a vertical cord. These muscles are rotated from side to side and it is this movement of the muscles and ligaments which causes the nerves to send a different kind of stimulation to the chakras. Nauli has a powerful effect on the physical body and is especially beneficial for the awakening of manipura chakra. Therefore, in this series the order of practice is: agnisar, then uddiyana and finally nauli.

TECHNIQUES

What are the different types of nauli?

Swami Niranjanananda: Nauli has four stages:

1. *Madhyama nauli*, in which both the rectus abdominis muscles overlying the stomach and intestines are contracted so that they form a prominent arch down the centre of the abdomen.

2. *Vama nauli*, in which the abdominal muscles on the left side of the abdominal wall are isolated and contracted.

3. *Dakshina nauli*, in which the abdominal muscles on the right side of the abdominal wall are isolated and contracted.

These three practices are done separately one after the other and complement each other. After practising agnisara and uddiyana bandha, and perfecting madhyama nauli, vama and dakshina nauli become easier. When complete mastery is gained over all three stages, the fourth type of nauli can be learnt.

4. *Bhramara nauli*, in which the abdominal muscles are progressively rotated and contracted. The three preceding practices are combined in this fourth variation called bhramara nauli or simply nauli. It has two parts: progressively contracting the muscles in a clockwise direction (circular rotation from right to left) and then doing the same in the opposite direction (circular rotation from left to right). Each rotation is completed five to ten times, according to individual capacity.

What is the role of nauli in other shatkarmas?

Swami Satyananda: Nauli is an integral part of basti and vastra dhauti, which are important shatkarmas.

Can nauli be used in shankhaprakshalana instead of the five asanas?

Swami Niranjanananda: Nauli is related to the digestive functions. The benefits of nauli are gained to some extent when one does *shankhaprakshalana*, washing of the intestines, or *laghoo shankhaprakshalana*, short intestinal wash. Although nauli is not practised at that time, the asanas used during shankhaprakshalana provide similar movement. Whether the five asanas of shankhaprakshalana or only nauli are practised, the benefit and effect is the same. Due to the stomach being bloated with water it is difficult to practise nauli during shankhaprakshalana, so Swami Satyananda replaced nauli with these five asanas, making it more scientific and accessible.

There is traction in *tadasana*, palm tree pose, which opens up the knots of the intestines and stomach. *Tiryak tadasana*, swaying palm tree pose, allows the water to swish from side to side, and *kati chakrasana*, waist rotating pose, squeezes the water down. In *tiryak bhujangasana*, twisting cobra pose, a supine posture, lateral pressure is created, after having created vertical pressure previously. *Udarakarshanasana*, abdominal stretch pose, a squatting posture, is more like nauli itself, as the stomach region is compressed, forcing and squeezing the water out.

The effect of nauli is similar to these asanas as in the perfection of nauli there are three movements. One movement is pulling the stomach in, as in uddiyana bandha, when one creates downward and upward pressure. The second movement is the lateral movement of the muscles, which is like swishing the water. The third is a vertical, up and down movement of the diaphragm, which again creates a downward pressure.

GUIDELINES FOR PRACTICE

How does one prepare for the practice of nauli?

Swami Satyananda: Nauli should be learned stage by stage and one should never attempt or expect to master it in one day.

As preparation, agnisara kriya and uddiyana bandha must first be mastered, then madhyama nauli, dakshina nauli and vama nauli. Madhyama nauli means to isolate the rectus abdominis in the centre. Dakshina nauli means isolation of the same in the right corner of the abdomen. Vama nauli means isolation in the left corner of the abdomen. These techniques should be learned either in the presence of an adept or through audio visual methods. In *Hatharatnavali* (1:34) the technique is described:

> *Idayaavartavegena tathaa pingalayaa punah.*
> *Ubhaabhyaam bhraamayeshchaishaahyantaraa keertitaa mayaa.*

> Fast rotation from ida and then again from pingala;
> Rotation of these two is called antara nauli according to me.

How should one prepare for the practice of nauli?

Swami Niranjanananda: It is essential to perfect agnisara kriya and uddiyana bandha prior to nauli kriya, otherwise nauli kriya is extremely difficult to perform.

Perfection of pranayama, especially mastery of external breath retention, is essential, as nauli cannot be practised for a lengthy duration until external breath retention is mastered.

How can the body's posture be adjusted to make nauli easier for beginners?

Swami Sivananda: When beginners do dakshina nauli, they should slightly bend towards the left side, and contract the left muscles. When they do vama nauli, they should bend a little to the right side. In madhyama nauli, all the muscles are pushed forward by contracting the two sides.

Is obesity an obstacle to the practice of nauli?

Swami Sivananda: This exercise is not possible for those who have a barrel-like belly. When it is difficult to carry one's own belly, one cannot even dream of success in this kriya. They must try by slow, gradual practice. For success, they will have to do hard and rigorous practice for a long time. Those who have a tender body, however, can easily learn and perform this kriya in a beautiful and efficient manner.

What are the obstacles to practising nauli?

Swami Satyananda: It is difficult for those who have a fat belly. It is excellent for those who have a slim body and a tender stomach and abdomen. Nauli should be performed with absolute care and precaution.

Nauli should never be practised when there is constipation or a loose stomach. It should not be practised in a hurry, but slowly and gradually. In the beginning it is advisable to practise it in the presence of a guru. Although the chances of mishap are rare, sometimes a wrong manipulation may create a knot or twist which will prove harmful. People suffering from piles should never do nauli. In this case, moola bandha and ashwini mudra are more helpful.

Nauli should never be practised in instances of fever which has no apparent cause, tuberculosis, bad breath or any infection. If any reactions take place or loose motions of the bowel ensue, the practice should be stopped immediately. Loose motion is actually an indication of irritation of the intestines. Constipation is the loss of the usual curvature of the intestine, resulting in undue pressure on wrong points of the colon.

When should nauli be practised?

Swami Niranjanananda: Nauli kriya should be undertaken only on an empty stomach. The ideal time is in the morning before breakfast. Otherwise it can be done at least five or six hours after eating.

How often and for how long should nauli be practised?

Swami Satyananda: There is no hard and fast rule as to the frequency and duration of practice for this kriya. The general recommendation is daily practice in the early morning for between twenty seconds and one minute on an empty stomach.

At first one should not do too many rounds. When trying to master madhyama nauli, five or six rounds is more than sufficient. With practice, a maximum of about ten rounds can be performed. When trying to master vama and dakshina nauli, three to five rounds each is sufficient. There should be no straining under any circumstances. One must pay attention to one's body and stop if there is any feeling of tiredness.

Once the practice of nauli is commenced, it should be continued regularly. If it is practised for an extended period of time and then suddenly stopped, the intestines lose their tone and the peristaltic movement becomes sluggish. Strong and healthy intestines are a valuable asset, which can prolong the lifespan. Therefore, this kriya should not be treated lightly. Even as a wrestler strengthens his body by gradually lifting weights, the yogi should strengthen his abdomen by slowly increasing the practice of nauli.

How many rounds of nauli should be practised?

Swami Niranjanananda: For a beginner, five or six rounds of madhyama nauli are sufficient. Gradually the number of rounds can be increased to ten, as long as there is no strain. Vama and dakshina nauli should be performed together, five to ten rounds each. Begin with five to ten rounds of bhramara nauli and slowly increase to twenty five over a period of months as more control is gained over the muscles.

What precautions should one be aware of when practising nauli kriya?

Swami Satyananda: If any pain is felt in the abdomen during nauli one should immediately stop the practice and try nauli the following day or when the pain subsides. If the pain persists seek proper guidance from an experienced yoga teacher or doctor.

When is nauli kriya contra-indicated?

Swami Niranjanananda: People who are recovering from major or abdominal surgery, or suffering from high blood pressure, hypertension, heart disease, hernia, gallstones or peptic ulcer should not practise nauli kriya. Those with abdominal complaints should consult a qualified specialist prior to practising nauli. Nauli kriya should not be practised during pregnancy. It can be practised five to six months after delivery to make the abdominal and pelvic muscles strong and healthy and to assist in the subtle realignment of internal organs.

BENEFITS

Why should nauli kriya be practised?

Swami Sivananda: Nauli kriya is intended for regenerating, invigorating and stimulating the abdominal organs and the gastrointestinal system. Nauli kriya eradicates chronic constipation, dyspepsia and all other diseases of the gastrointestinal system. The liver and pancreas are toned, and the kidneys and other organs of the abdomen function properly.

Nauli is an ideal pick-me-up, and a blessing to humanity. If the yogic exercises are done in the right way with the right mental attitude, they lead to spiritual growth. In *Hatharatnavali* (1:33) it is written:

Tundaargni sandeepana paachanaadi sandeepikaanandakaree sadaiva.
Ashesha doshaamayashoshanee cha hathakriyaamauliriyam cha naulih.

Nauli, the crown of hatha practices, makes the gastric fire blaze up, improves digestion etc., invariably brings a feeling of wellbeing and completely destroys all disorders and diseases.

What are the health benefits of nauli kriya?

Swami Satyananda: Nauli increases the general vitality of the whole body. It removes abdominal disorders and strengthens intestinal peristalsis. It checks and restores intestinal flexibility and tone.

Nauli is a beneficial practice for women and does not interfere with the reproductive functions. The correct practice of nauli may rectify a displaced uterus; madhyama nauli is beneficial for the condition where the uterus is slightly tilted.

Nauli kriya sets right disorders of the stomach, and rectifies any weakness in the peristaltic movements. Worms of the stomach and intestines can also be expelled by the practice of nauli. Nauli helps alleviate diabetes by improving the efficiency of the pancreas and improves blood circulation. It prevents hernia, which is caused by weak and inefficient abdominal muscles. Nauli strengthens these muscles, thereby preventing the occurrence of hernia. If one already suffers from hernia, nauli should not be practised.

Other shatkarmas and asanas stimulate the digestion, but nauli is said to be the best for this. It quickly tones the abdominal muscles, nerves, intestines, reproductive, excretory and urinary organs: the entire internal system is stimulated by this practice. When the abdominal muscles are manipulated, not only are they toned, but all the internal organs are massaged. In *Hatha Yoga Pradipika* (2:34) it states:

Mandaagnisandeepanapaachanaadisandhaapikaananda-karee sadaiva.
Asheshadoshaamayashoshanee cha hathakriyaa mauliriyam cha naulih.

Nauli is foremost of the hatha yoga practices. It kindles the digestive fire, removing indigestion, sluggish digestion, and all disorders of the doshas, and brings about happiness.

Asana and pranayama practice definitely generate energy, but nauli activates the system in a much shorter time and with greater force. Its effects are particularly noticeable on the digestive and excretory systems. It generates heat in the body, stimulates digestion, assimilation and absorption, thereby reducing excretion. It balances the endocrine system and helps control the production of sex hormones.

Nauli speeds up blood circulation and reduces blood stagnation. It is especially useful for alleviating constipation, indigestion, nervous diarrhoea, acidity, flatulence, depression, hormonal imbalances, sexual and urinary disorders, laziness, dullness, lack of energy and emotional disturbances. Its practice helps with control of the appetite and sensual desires. Nauli also strengthens the willpower. With these attainments, the practitioner will definitely find deeper satisfaction within.

Why is nauli an important practice for both the physical and pranic bodies?

Swami Niranjanananda: In the practice of nauli the muscles of the abdominal wall are contracted and brought to the midline where they form a central contour about ten centimetres long. When nauli is perfected, apart from this contour, the abdomen is so flat that the practitioner can literally count the bones of the vertebral column. In this state, pressure is exerted on the stomach and intestines. All the organs of the abdomen and stomach are massaged. The abdominal muscles become strong and healthy, reducing the risk of hernia (the protrusion of tissue through a weakness in the muscular wall). Bowel function is improved and constipation reduced. The pancreas is energized and insulin is secreted, making nauli particularly beneficial for diabetics. The digestive fire is activated.

It is clear that nauli influences the physical, mental and pranic consciousness. Tissues throughout the body, such as muscles, blood vessels, endocrine glands and the nervous system, are subtly purified. Nauli rejuvenates the pranic energy within the whole body, which in turn enhances the efficiency of the brain.

What are the effects of nauli on the pranic body?

Swami Satyananda: During nauli, suction takes place, causing apana to be drawn upwards and joined with prana at the navel. This creates yogic heat, which influences the quality of one's meditation, thinking and decisions. Nauli is intended for those who wish to practise higher yoga.

Nauli is the most important shatkarma practice. The practice of nauli is intended to recharge or awaken the naval centre, the *manipura chakra* which is important in laya yoga. Nauli has a direct influence on the manipura chakra trigger point, or *kshetram*. Manipura is the centre of energy distribution, both gross and subtle, in the whole body. Nauli helps to remove blockages in the energy flows of the body. This leads to better health and more energy. Indirectly, nauli helps to increase mental clarity and power by harmonizing the energy flows in the body.

Why is nauli an important practice for manipura chakra?

Swami Niranjanananda: In kundalini yoga and hatha yoga, the practice of nauli is undertaken to influence and awaken the *chakras*, psychic centres. In the physical body there are nerve plexuses, or networks, at the places where the chakras are located. These nerve plexuses, corresponding to the chakras, have branches that extend throughout the body. The effect of nauli is felt on these nerve plexuses.

Nauli is practised to clear manipura chakra of impurities and to remove the blocks in the channels of pranic force. The main pranic currents are brought into a specific position which is conducive to the awakening of manipura chakra. As such, nauli plays a significant role in awakening manipura chakra.

Why is nauli fourth in the sequence of the shatkarmas in *Gheranda Samhita*?

Swami Niranjanananda: In the sequence of shatkarmas in *Gheranda Samhita*, nauli has been given fourth place. There is a reason for this. The first need is to purify the body, ridding it of disorders. Therefore, the first three shatkarmas – dhauti, basti and neti – purify and remove defects from the internal organs, using water, air or some solid object. Internal toxins and waste products are thus removed, and internal defects or imbalanced doshas are rectified.

The purpose of the next three shatkarma practices – nauli/lauliki, kapalbhati and trataka – is also purification of the body, but their process is different. These three practices are undertaken only after the body has been purified internally. After purification, the need of the body is energy.

With the practice of nauli kriya, the body is sensitized, strong vibrations are created in the pranic body and mental concentration is achieved, allowing the consciousness to quickly move from one state to another. Nauli activates the digestive fire, as does the third practice of antar dhauti, vahnisara kriya, now more widely known as agnisara kriya. While nauli and agnisara appear similar, their benefits differ markedly. Agnisara kriya is a preliminary stage, whereas lauliki, or nauli kriya, is a stage of awakening and attainment.

10

Kapalbhati: Frontal Brain Cleansing

WHAT IS KAPALBHATI?

What is kapalbhati?

Swami Satyananda: The last of the six shatkarmas in *Hatha Yoga Pradipika* and *Gheranda Samhita* is kapalbhati. *Kapala* means the 'cranium' or 'forehead'. *Bhati* is 'light' or 'splendour', but it also means 'perception and knowledge'. Kapalbhati is a pranayama technique which invigorates the entire brain and awakens the dormant centres which are responsible for subtle perception. In English it is called the 'frontal brain cleansing' technique. *Hatha Yoga Pradipika* (2:35) describes the way of breathing as being like a bellows:

> *Bhastraavallohakaarasya rechapoorau sasambhramau.*
> *Kapaalabhaatirvikhyaataa kaphadoshavishoshanee.*
>
> Perform exhalation and inhalation rapidly like the bellows (of a blacksmith). This is called kapalbhati; it destroys all mucous disorders.

Kapalbhati is a similar practice to bhastrika pranayama except that exhalation is emphasized and inhalation is the result of forcing the air out. In normal breathing, inhalation is active and exhalation is passive. Kapalbhati reverses that process so that exhalation becomes active and inhalation passive. This is like the pumping action of the blacksmith's bellows; when the bellows are closed the air is pushed out, and when they are opened the air is sucked in due to the vacuum effect that is created. Similarly, when one inhales in kapalbhati, it should be a reaction to the forced exhalation.

Why is kapalbhati classed as a shatkarma when it is a pranayama technique?

Swami Satyananda: Kapalbhati is a shatkarma, but it is also a pranayama. Whereas other pranayamas require a somewhat purified system, kapalbhati does not, as it purifies; so it comes under the shatkarmas.

Why is kapalbhati the sixth shatkarma in *Gheranda Samhita*?

Swami Niranjanananda: In *Gheranda Samhita* the first five groups of shatkarmas: dhauti, basti, neti, nauli and trataka, aim to cleanse or purify the organs of the body, and to achieve mental concentration and stability. The sixth shatkarma, kapalbhati, is for the purification of pranamaya kosha. It has also been known as bhalbhati, but kapalbhati is now a more common name. *Kapala* means 'skull', *bhal* means 'forehead'. In *Gheranda Samhita* (1:55) three types of kapalbhati are named:

> *Vaatakramena vyutkramena sheetkramena visheshatah;*
> *Bhaalabhaatim tridhaa kuryaatkaphadosham nivaarayet.*
>
> Vatakrama, vyutkrama and sheetkrama are the three types of bhalbhati. Practising them eliminates phlegm and mucus from the body.

Sage Gheranda discusses three practices which are all variations of bhalbhati or kapalbhati. The first, *vatakrama*, uses air. The second and third, *vyutkrama* and *sheetkrama* use water in a manner similar to jala neti.

What is the difference between bhastrika and kapalbhati?

Swami Sivananda: In bhastrika *kumbhaka*, retention of breath, is practised at the end of the required rounds. In kapalbhati, however, there is no kumbhaka. In kapalbhati, inhalation is long and mild, while exhalation is quick and forceful. In bhastrika, inhalation is done as quickly as exhalation. This is the only difference between kapalbhati and bhastrika. In kapalbhati, exhalation should be done forcibly and quickly by contracting the abdominal muscles with a backward push.

What is the difference between hatha yoga and raja yoga kapalbhati?

Swami Satyananda: There are two ways of practising kapalbhati. The method of a hatha yogi is to simply expel the breath with force, whereas a raja yogi takes his awareness to *chidakasha*, the mind space, after the final expulsion. This additional practice removes certain cerebral tensions. Just as an expeller removes bad air from a room, even so the brain is shaken by the process of kapalbhati.

What are the different kapalbhati techniques within the hatha yoga tradition?

Swami Niranjanananda: *Gheranda Samhita* describes three types of kapalbhati: two use water, one uses air. The form using air is named *vatakrama kapalbhati.* It resembles the practice given in Hatha Yoga Pradipika, although the techniques are slightly different.

The major difference between the method of kapalbhati in the two traditions is that in the *Hatha Yoga Pradipika* of Yogi Swatmarama, there is no mention of breathing through alternate nostrils. It can be assumed that this is a preparation for Yogi Swatmarama's version of bhastrika pranayama. As with other shatkarmas, Yogi Swatmarama seems to deal with the shatkarmas at a more introductory level than Sage Gheranda.

Hatharatnavali (1:54–55) describes kapalbhati performed both with and without alternating the nostrils:

> *Atha kapaalabhaatih*
> *Bhastrivallauhakaaraanaam rechapoorasusambhramau.*
> *Kapaalabhaatirvikhyaataa sarvarogavishoshanee.*
>
> *Kapaalam bhraamayetsavyamapasavyam tu vegatah.*
> *Rechapoorvakamuktena kapaalabhaatiruchyate.*
>
> Now kapalabhati: Rapid performance of inhalation and exhalation like the bellows of the blacksmith is kapalbhati, well known as the destroyer of all diseases. (54)
>
> Fast rotation of breathing from left to right and right to left, and exhalation and inhalation is called kapalbhati. (55)

What is involved in the practice of vatakrama kapalbhati?

Swami Niranjanananda: Vatakrama kapalbhati is described in *Gheranda Samhita* as one of the cleansing practices. As it uses air to clean the nasal area, it is also considered to be a type of pranayama. After inhaling, the air is expelled quickly, just as a blacksmith firing a furnace expels air from his bellows. On inhalation, air is allowed to enter the body passively, at a normal speed. In *Gheranda Samhita* (1:56–57) instructions are given:

> *Idayaa poorayedvaayum rechayetpingalayaa punah;*
> *Pingalayaa poorayitvaa punashchandrena rechayet.*
>
> *Poorakam rechakam kritvaa vegena na tu dhaarayet;*
> *Evamabhyaasa yogena kapha dosham nivaarayet.*
>
> The breath is to be inhaled through ida nadi (the left nostril) and exhaled through pingala nadi (the right nostril). Then the breath is inhaled through surya nadi (the right nostril) and exhaled through chandra nadi (the left nostril). (56)
>
> Inhalation and exhalation should be fast; do not hold it. This technique removes kapha dosha. (57)

Vatakrama kapalbhati is a difficult practice, as along with the forced exhalation, energy is focused through only one nostril at a time. Also, in this practice, awareness is taken to the forehead on exhalation, rather than to the abdomen as is usually the case in this type of vitalizing pranayama.

How does vatakrama kapalbhati benefit the respiratory system?

Swami Niranjanananda: With the practice of vatakrama kapalbhati fresh air reaches the lower peripheries of the lungs, while stale air is expelled. During this practice the respiratory system is activated, and the exchange of oxygen and carbon dioxide is increased. This practice benefits people suffering from respiratory ailments, including chronic bronchitis and tuberculosis.

People suffering from severe asthma and chronic lung disease often develop a habit of using the accessory muscles of respiration to breathe forcibly, and also tend to exhale with increased muscular force, making the muscles tired and causing fatigue. Such people should practise kapalbhati, but not while having an asthma attack.

What effect does vatakrama kapalbhati have on the brain?

Swami Niranjanananda: In the normal breathing process, the muscles of respiration – the diaphragm and intercostal muscles – actively contract during inhalation. During exhalation they generally relax passively: one has to make an effort to breathe in, whereas no effort is required for exhalation. Vatakrama kapalbhati reverses this natural process – the exhalation requires effort and is active, while the inhalation is natural or passive. This causes different neuronal pathways within the brain to fire and thus helps to awaken dormant brain centres.

Vatakrama kapalbhati increases cardiac output. With the increased blood flow, the frontal brain is purified and becomes more active. At the subtle level, prana shakti flows more strongly in this region of the brain. As well as bringing about improvement in the respiratory system and abdomen, vatakrama kapalbhati is one of the best practices for purification of this frontal part of the brain. It is a powerful technique for making the mind peaceful and aware.

How does vatakrama kapalbhati benefit the abdominal region?

Swami Niranjanananda: Vatakrama kapalbhati activates the muscles involved in exhalation, mainly the abdominal muscles, thus increasing the blood flow to them. At the same time, the digestive organs are activated, massaged and strengthened.

What is the effect of vatakrama kapalbhati on one's energy?

Swami Niranjanananda: After practising ten rounds of kapalbhati, one does not feel like sleeping. People who become tired after doing mental work, or who go to sleep or feel like sleeping after getting up in the morning find kapalbhati beneficial.

What is vyutkrama kapalbhati?

Swami Niranjanananda: Vyutkrama kapalbhati is similar to jala neti. In vyutkrama water is taken in through the nose, held in the throat and then expelled through the mouth. As in jala neti, after the water cleanses the nasal passages, not only the nostrils but the throat and the pharynx, the area behind the nose and mouth, are cleansed. This technique is described in *Gheranda Samhita* (1:58):

> *Naasaabhyaam jalamaakrishya punarvaktrena rechayet;*
> *Paayam paayam vyutkramena shleshmaadosham nivaarayet.*
>
> Suck water through both nostrils and expel it through the mouth. Practise this repeatedly. This vyutkrama kapalbhati removes kapha disorders.

What is the effect of vyutkrama kapalbhati on bindu chakra?

Swami Niranjanananda: When water enters the mouth via the nose, it touches certain nerves which generally do not come into contact with water or the tongue. If there is an attempt to touch the nasopharynx, the area behind the nostrils, by folding the tongue backwards in khechari mudra, usually the tongue is not able to reach it. In general, only the flow of the breath reaches this point. When the tongue does touch that region, in perfected khechari mudra, the sensation created by this contact awakens bindu chakra.

It is said that after perfecting khechari mudra, nectar flows from bindu and one drinks nectar. The practice of vyutkrama is recommended for those people who cannot gain mastery over khechari mudra. It stimulates the nadis which lie in the region of the nasopharynx and bindu visarga is awakened to some extent. The awakening of bindu does not necessarily mean that nectar will start dripping. It takes time, as there are some centres in the body that are extremely sensitive and activated by any kind of touch, but there are other centres that need constant pressure. The centre which secretes nectar and brings it down from bindu is truly awakened only by the pressure of khechari mudra.

What is sheetkrama kapalbhati?

Swami Niranjanananda: The third practice of bhalbati given in *Gheranda Samhita* (1:59) is sheetkrama kapalbhati, in which water is sucked in through the mouth and expelled through the nose. *Sheetkritya peetvaa vaktrena naasaanaalarvirechayet,* here *sheetkritya* means breathing in deeply making a sound, and sucking water inside.

While doing sheetkrama, the tongue is curled, creating a channel inside the mouth. This part of the practice is reminiscent of sheetali pranayama. Suction is created so that water enters the mouth via the curled tongue. The water is held in the mouth and then expelled in small amounts through the nose every few seconds. A second small amount of water is then taken in through the mouth and expelled. In this way water is slowly expelled through the nose in small amounts, with each expulsion lasting one second.

What are the benefits and effects of sheetkrama kapalbhati?

Swami Niranjanananda: This practice has many benefits. *Gheranda Samhita* (1:59–60) describes them in brief:

> *Sheetkritya peetvaa vaktrena naasaanaalarvirechayet;*
> *Evamabhyaasayogena kaamadeva samo bhavet.*
>
> *Na jaayate vaarddhakam cha jvaro naiva prajaayate;*
> *Bhavetsvachchhanda dehashcha kapha dosham nivaarayet.*
>
> Suck in water through the mouth with a hissing sound and expel it through the nose. Through this practice the body of the practitioner becomes as beautiful as that of Kamadeva, the god of love. (59)
>
> Signs of old age do not manifest. Cleanliness and purity manifest in the body and kapha dosha is removed. (60)

Evamabhyaasayogena kaamadeva samo bhavet, means that by doing this practice a person starts looking like Kamadeva, the god of love, known in the West as Cupid. One becomes healthy as impurities of the body are removed and the face glows. A person who perfects this practice is not marked by disease or old age. When a person is healthy, fewer wrinkles appear. A truly healthy person will have a happy life even in old age, but an unhealthy person feels frail even when young.

From a scientific angle, the condition described here is one of ideal health. When the body becomes completely free from internal disorders, when the negative effects of the doshas described in ayurveda do not remain, and when the mind is peaceful and steady, real health is attained. This achievement is not only physical, but also mental.

Sage Gheranda points out the use of this cleansing technique for attaining good health and beauty. This is, however, only a side effect, the reason for the practice is the awakening of bindu visarga. When bindu is awakened and the nectar of immortality, *amrita*, flows, the body becomes lustrous.

GUIDELINES FOR PRACTICE

How many rounds of kapalbhati can be safely practised?

Swami Satyananda: In kapalbhati a greater number of respirations can be taken than in bhastrika pranayama, as hyperventilation does not occur. Up to two hundred breaths can be taken after months of practice, unless advised otherwise by one's guru.

If dizziness is experienced while practising, it means the breathing is too forceful. If this occurs, the practice should be stopped and recommenced after a few minutes of quiet sitting. When it is resumed, it should be done with more awareness and less force. There should not be a feeling of breathlessness before completing the round.

Is kapalbhati practised through the nose or the mouth?

Swami Niranjanananda: For the entire practice breathing should be through the nose, not the mouth. If the nose is blocked, jala neti should be performed beforehand.

Where should the awareness be held during kapalbhati?

Swami Niranjanananda: The mind should be fixed at chidakasha, the dark empty space inside the forehead. With the eyes closed, one looks into this space. The lungs should move like a bellows. One feels pranic vibrations in chidakasha, and also feels that the frontal part of the brain is being purified.

When should kapalbhati be practised and for how long?

Swami Niranjanananda: Kapalbhati should be done after asana or neti, and just before concentration or meditation. It should not be practised at night, as it will cause difficulty sleeping.

Experienced practitioners with a strong and pure body can do this practice for hours at a time, but in general not more than ten to twenty rounds are recommended. Beginners should do two to three rounds only. After some weeks the number of rounds can be increased one at a time.

When is kapalbhati contra-indicated?

Swami Niranjanananda: If any feelings of unwellness are experienced, the practice should be stopped. It should not be practised in extremely hot weather, or when one is dehydrated, or suffering from irritability or anger. Although kapalbhati can be adapted so that it is helpful during labour, it is not recommended during pregnancy without expert guidance.

Kapalbhati should not be undertaken by people suffering from high blood pressure, heart problems, ulcers, fever, constipation, hernia, anger or excessive restlessness.

BENEFITS

What are the health benefits of practising kapalbhati?

Swami Sivananda: Kapalbhati cleanses the respiratory system and nasal passages, and removes spasm in the bronchial tubes. Consequently asthma is relieved and may be cured in the course of time. Tuberculosis may be cured by this practice. Impurities of the blood are thrown out. The apices of the lungs receive proper oxygenation and thereby do not afford a suitable breeding ground for bacteria.

The lungs are well developed by this practice. Carbon dioxide is largely eliminated, and the tissues and cells absorb a large quantity of oxygen. The heart functions properly. The circulatory and respiratory systems are toned, and the practitioner enjoys good health.

What are the general effects of kapalbhati on the body and mind?

Swami Satyananda: Kapalbhati is an excellent practice that purifies the frontal part of the brain, massages the abdominal organs and improves respiration.

Kapalbhati is also a powerful method of waking up the mind. The frontal lobes of the brain are cleared by speeding up the blood flow. At a more subtle level it also stimulates pranic flow in the same region. Therefore, if one has a lot of mental work to complete, but feels tired, the mind can be energized and made alert with a few rounds of kapalbhati. After ten rounds of kapalbhati it is impossible to sleep, so it can be used to energize the mind for mental work when one feels tired, and to remove sleepiness early in the morning. It is an ideal practice to do immediately before commencing meditation.

How does kapalbhati benefit the respiratory system?

Swami Satyananda: Kapalbhati benefits the respiratory system by cleaning out the lungs and improving their elasticity, resulting in more efficient oxygen-carbon dioxide exchange.

Kapalbhati should certainly be practised by those suffering from respiratory ailments such as bronchitis and tuberculosis. Those who suffer from asthma and emphysema will, from habit and necessity, use forceful exhalations to expel air from the lungs. This tends to induce severe muscular tiredness. Kapalbhati, practised at times other than during an attack, may be useful in making respiratory muscles stronger, as well as improving the general tone of the lungs.

How does kapalbhati prepare one for the practice of meditation?

Swami Satyananda: Kapalbhati is one of the best preparatory techniques for meditative practice. It empties the mind of thoughts, emotional feelings and excessive visions. It induces a tranquil, receptive state of mind. Experience has shown that the ideal meditation practice to follow kapalbhati is chidakasha dharana.

Why does kapalbhati energize the brain?

Swami Satyananda: Normal breathing is characterized by active contraction of the inspiratory muscles, such as the diaphragm and the external intercostals; expiration occurs passively on the cessation of this contraction of the internal intercostals. Kapalbhati reverses this process: exhalation is active and inhalation is passive. This induces a reversal in the flow of the nerve impulses to and from the brain, bringing about stimulation and awakening of the brain centres. This is one reason for the brain-stimulating effect of kapalbhati, at least physiologically. It should be noted that the expiratory muscles usually only come into action when there is obstruction to respiration, or when there is a great need for extra oxygen in the system.

Does the forced exhalation in kapalbhati have a direct effect on the brain?

Swami Satyananda: The effects of kapalbhati and bhastrika are similar, but due to the forced and longer exhalation, kapalbhati affects the brain differently. In his book, *Pranayama: The Yoga of Breathing* Andre van Lysebeth describes a physiological phenomenon in which, during normal inhalation, the fluid around the brain is compressed causing the brain to contract slightly. With exhalation this cerebrospinal fluid is decompressed and the brain slightly expands. This is the mechanical influence of the respiratory cycle on the brain itself. Forced exhalation in kapalbhati increases the massaging effect on the brain by enhancing the decompression effect on every exhalation.

The average number of breaths being fifteen per minute, the brain is compressed and decompressed that many times, but in kapalbhati, one is breathing fifty to one hundred times, stimulating the brain three to seven times more than normal per round. Kapalbhati also expels more carbon dioxide and other waste gases from the cells and lungs than normal breathing.

Why is kapalbhati practised before meditation?

Swami Niranjanananda: Kapalbhati is an ideal preparation for meditation: those wishing to progress in meditation should practise kapalbhati prior to meditating. Kapalbhati makes the mind peaceful and receptive, helping it to rise above emotions and become thoughtless. It is best to practise chidakasha dharana after kapalbhati.

Does kapalbhati help prepare the sadhaka for the safe awakening of kundalini?

Swami Niranjanananda: Hatha yogis believe that ida and pingala nadis are purified by doing kapalbhati. In kundalini yoga it is said that at times one nadi flows while at other times the other nadi flows. In general, the flow of breath in the nostrils, the *swara*, changes every ninety minutes. It alternates between the right nostril, which is associated with pingala nadi, and the left nostril, which is associated with ida nadi. When sushumna flows, prana moves freely through both nostrils at the same time. Only rarely, however, do both nadis flow simultaneously, but it can be experienced if there is awareness of the breathing process. However, when the flow of the breath is equal in both nostrils, it still cannot be assumed that both ida and pingala nadis are free from disorders; an equal flow of air in both nostrils just happens from time to time.

It has also been said in kundalini yoga that if a practitioner does not have control over the swara and nadis, then pure, stainless kundalini, free from any disorder, could rise through nadis that are disordered and impure. If kundalini starts rising through ida or pingala nadi the person will begin to have certain experiences such as extreme dullness or excitability, depending on the state of the nadi and which nadi is involved. Without sufficient preparation of body, mind and prana, sometimes the person may even become mad, losing body consciousness. However, if the cleansing process has been done properly, the rising of kundalini will be through the sushumna passage.

How does the practice of kapalbhati assist in awakening ajna chakra?

Swami Niranjanananda: It is not kapalbhati which awakens ajna, but the reaction which takes place when one is able to perform a pranayama practice correctly that helps to awaken various chakras. Kapalbhati stimulates the nerves; they in turn activate the nadis, which then activate the pranas; the pranas are attracted towards the region in the nervous system where activity is taking place, which in kapalbhati is the forehead.

There are moments when the body, mind and prana all reach their peak at the same time, like the biorhythms which are calculated from the date of birth. According to the yogic concept, there are physical, mental and pranic biorhythms. When these three waves reach a certain point, there is harmony in the different koshas. This harmony is experienced in the form of a clear mind, thought and expression; increased nervous, emotional and mental energies; good health, physical fitness and mental relaxation. The biorhythms undergo many changes in the course of daily activities. Knowledge of these rhythms at the time of kapalbhati practice makes one deeply aware of the pranic and mental states. Kapalbhati helps to control the mental state by influencing the physical level, by altering the experiences, the input and output of the nervous system and the brain, and speeding up the metabolism.

In the context of hatha yoga, kapalbhati is practised to achieve a totally one-pointed state of mind. For the sake of our understanding, the practice of kapalbhati may be compared to the state of pratyahara. In *pratyahara* one tries to divert the mind from external distractions and focus it at one point, and then in the practice of *dharana* one tries to intensify the concentration. In kapalbhati, like pratyahara, effort is made to relax the dissipation of the annamaya, manomaya and pranamaya koshas. The aim of kapalbhati is to awaken ajna chakra.

11

Trataka: Steady Gazing

UNDERSTANDING TRATAKA

What is trataka?

Swami Satyananda: The word *trataka* means 'steady gazing'. If someone is staring for a long time, that is trataka. The practice of trataka involves gazing at a point or object without winking or blinking the eyes. It is a method of focusing the eyes, and in turn the mind, on one point to the exclusion of all else. The object can be either external, which is called *bahir* or *bahiranga trataka*, outer gazing, or internal, which is called *antar*, or *antaranga trataka*, inner gazing. Bahiranga is simpler to practise as one simply gazes at an object or symbol, whereas antaranga trataka involves the clear and stable inner visualization of an object.

Trataka is one of the most direct, simple and effective techniques for attaining concentration of mind. It can be practised by everyone and the benefits are vast. By practising trataka, all the attention and power of the mind is channeled into one continuous stream, allowing latent potential to arise spontaneously.

In *Hatha Yoga Pradipika* (2:31) trataka is described:

Nireekshennishchaladrishaa sookshmalakshyam samaahitah.
Ashrusampaataparyantamaachaaryaistraatakam smritam.

> Looking intently with an unwavering gaze at a small point until tears are shed is known as trataka by the acharyas (teachers).

Yogi Swatmarama's instruction is to gaze at a small point, *sukshma lakshyam*. *Sukshma* can mean 'small' or 'subtle'. In the practice of trataka an object is gazed at until its subtle form manifests in front of the closed eyes.

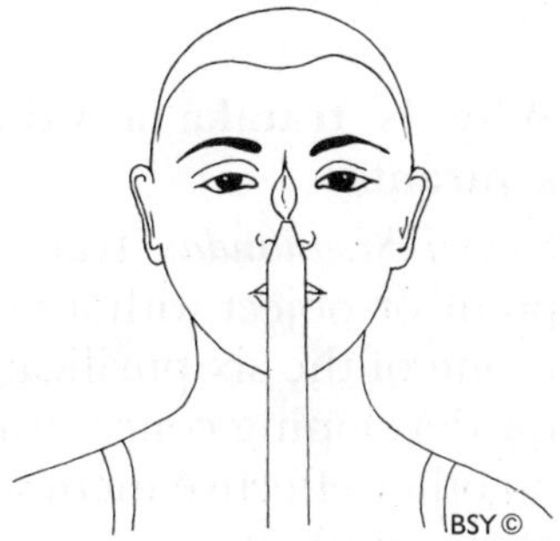

Trataka

The best object is the flame of the candle. The flame is looked at for some time, then the eyes are closed and one tries to see the candle inside. It is not imagination, it is the effect of the light on the brain and ocular system. The candle remains burning inside, one concentrates on it, and the mind becomes introverted.

What is the process of trataka?

Swami Sivananda: Trataka is a hatha yoga shatkarma which also plays a prominent part in raja yoga and jnana yoga. Trataka is the focusing of one's energy towards an object, a thing, or an idea; one then observes every detail of it, dissecting, analyzing, consciously and subconsciously drawing to oneself every possible bit of information regarding the object, both within and without.

What is involved in trataka?

Swami Niranjanananda: Trataka means to gaze at a fixed point with steady vision. Theoretically, there are three elements in trataka: the first is the viewer seated in the place of practice, the second is the object in front of the viewer, and the third is the process of gazing. When there is steady awareness of these three elements, one has entered a state of one-pointed internal consciousness. Trataka is described in *Gheranda Samhita* (1:53):

Nimeshonmeshakam tyaktvaa sookshmalakshyam nireekshayet;
Patanti yaavadashrooni traatakam prochyate budhaih.

Gazing at a subtle object without blinking the eyes, until tears begin to fall, is known as trataka.

Why is trataka a valuable practice for all spiritual aspirants?

Swami Sivananda: Trataka is steady gazing at a particular point or object without winking or blinking. Although this is one of the six purificatory exercises, it is mainly intended for developing concentration and mental focusing. There is no other effective method for the control of the mind. Some of the students who claim to belong to jnana yoga neglect important exercises such as this one, because it is described as hatha yoga.

Therefore, once again I say that bhakti yoga, jnana yoga, hatha yoga, karma yoga, etc., are not incompatibles like cocaine and soda bicarbonate. They are not antagonistic to each other. Many people benefit from this useful exercise. It is useful for students of hatha yoga, jnana yoga, bhakti yoga and raja yoga. When the most suitable method is selected, the spiritual benefits are definately realized.

Ramana Maharshi, the famous jnani of Tiruvannamalai, used to do this exercise. If one went to his ashram for darshan, his practice of trataka could be clearly seen. While seated on the sofa in his room, he used to gaze at the walls. When he sat on the veranda in an easy chair, he looked steadily at the distant hills or the sky. This enabled him to keep a balanced state of mind. Nothing could distract his mind. He was always calm and cool. He was not distracted at all by anyone, even though his bhaktas might be talking and singing by his side.

Trataka should not be neglected for the mere reason that it comes under hatha yoga. Even though a seeker may claim to be a student of jnana yoga or bhakti yoga, trataka should be taken up. It is an effective and powerful remedy for a wandering mind, and undoubtedly prepares the mind for perfection of dhyana and samadhi. Trataka is surely a means to an end and the yogic ladder must be ascended step by step.

When does trataka become a raja yoga practice?

Swami Niranjanananda: In the classical hatha yoga texts, trataka is described as one of the six shatkarmas, or cleansing techniques. It also acts as a stepping stone between the physically-oriented and mentally-oriented techniques which lead to higher awareness. In this sense trataka forms a bridge between hatha yoga and raja yoga. When trataka is practised until the tears roll down, it is part of hatha yoga, when practised with inner visualization, it is part of raja yoga.

Why is trataka the final shatkarma?

Swami Niranjanananda: Trataka is one of the cleansing or purification techniques of hatha yoga. Most people know the simple version of this technique, and believe that trataka means to gaze at something continuously. It is also believed that by practising trataka the eyes develop a magnetic quality by which anyone can be hypnotized and any type of siddhi can be achieved.

In yoga, however, the practice of trataka is not seen as a technique for achieving siddhis, but as a process of purification, one of the shatkarmas. First, using neti, dhauti and basti, an effort is made to purify the body by removing toxic elements. Then, in lauliki, or nauli kriya, the aim is to bring the subtle aspects of the physical body under control. Finally, with the practices of kapalbhati and trataka an effort is made to cleanse and calm the brain.

How is trataka practised in tantra?

Swami Satyananda: Tantra, probably the most all-inclusive spiritual system ever developed and the root of yoga, includes wide-ranging practise of trataka, whether using yantras, deities or objects as the focus of worship or awareness.

How is trataka used in other spiritual systems?

Swami Satyananda: The practice of trataka is used in one form or another by almost every religious and spiritual system, though often heavily disguised. In Hinduism it is an integral part of religious practice to sit in front of a picture or the statue of a deity and concentrate on it. Although this is regarded as a form of worship, it is actually a form of trataka, for the aim is to concentrate the mind on the external deity. From this practice the devotee obtains mental peace and a meditative state. Furthermore, the ability to create internal visualizations at will is developed, so that inner trataka can be practised.

In the *Uddhava Gita*, Sri Krishna instructs his disciple Uddhava in this form of trataka: "Having withdrawn the senses (pratyahara) from contact with the surroundings, the devotee should concentrate on my form, especially one part such as my smiling face. Then he should be aware of my all-pervading self which is free like the sky. Leaving that after some time, he should feel as though he is one with me, and stop thinking of all other things. He will see me, the *antaryamin*, inner being, in himself, and himself in me like the light that is united with the fire. All doubts about matter, knowledge and action will completely cease."

Trataka is also practised in Christianity, although in a less obvious manner. In every church there are idols of Christ, candles and the symbolic cross. These objects act as focal points for trataka, although of course, it is not known by that name. All of these forms have a deep-rooted symbolic meaning which generally acts below the level of normal awareness; these symbols correlate with and stimulate experiences and memories that are contained in what Jung called the collective unconscious. Therefore, these objects of awareness invoke experiences and knowledge of which one is normally unaware.

In Tibetan Buddhism, trataka is often practised on various deities, yantras and mandalas. Even Zen Buddhism uses trataka in the form of staring at a blank wall. The practice of trataka is universal and has been used throughout the ages as a method of transcending normal experience. It is simple yet extremely powerful, which is why so many different systems use it as a means for spiritual upliftment.

What do trataka, yoga nidra and hypnosis have in common?

Swami Niranjanananda: The ultimate object of all these techniques is the same but the actual techniques are different. The common aim of yoga nidra, trataka and hypnosis is developing the faculties and stopping the dissipation of the mind. When one is able to stop the dissipated nature of the mind it becomes possible to go deep within and awaken the faculties of the subconscious and unconscious mind.

How are pratyahara and dharana experienced during trataka?

Swami Niranjanananda: Trataka falls into two groups: pratyahara and dharana. Trataka aims to control the dissipation that occurs when one becomes aware of form. Form is seen by everyone and that form is recognized as something that is visible to everyone. That form symbolizes the state of mental dissipation.

Pratyahara trataka involves gazing at an external point, whether a candle, symbol, yantra or mandala. The eyes are considered to be the most active sensory field. The eyes are constantly looking at things; looking at so many things means that there is not actually awareness of everything that is seen, and only the information that the mind acknowledges is recognized. To have control over these visual perceptions and channel the impressions received through them is the aim of trataka – control over the aspect of form, the awareness of form. Through pratyahara trataka the sense of sight is concentrated on one object, to the exclusion of all else. This focus is so powerful that the other senses also lose their externalized nature, becoming quiet and still. The state of pratyahara is experienced.

Another form of trataka is antar or inner trataka. It is a simple method of concentration or *dharana*. The process is similar to outer trataka, but instead of using an external aid on which to focus the visual perception, one develops and awakens one's internal visual perceptions. The simple act of holding the image in the mind for an extended period of time helps to focus the dissipated energies of the senses, intellect and emotions at one point.

This acute or undivided concentration in which one is able to focus the mind wilfully, first of all on a manifest object and later on some concept or idea, is the purpose of trataka. It provides an unfluctuating and unwavering state of mind. The mental storehouse of visual impressions is released through the development of this technique.

TECHNIQUES

In trataka, can an image be created at the heart centre instead of in chidakash?

Swami Satyananda: Although trataka is usually described as a technique in which one creates the image in front of the eyes, there is absolutely no reason why one should not mentally create a picture at the heart centre. Many of the ancient yogic texts recommend this place for creation of the image. In the *Kathopanishad* it says that one can create an inner image at the heart. One must therefore experiment and find the best object and the best location. One shouldn't feel limited to the objects and techniques that are usually given, as they are only intended as a guide.

What are the different techniques for practising trataka?

Swami Niranjanananda: Trataka consists of six different modes of practice:

1. *Bahya drishti*, outer trataka, which is also known as *bahiranga trataka* or *bahir trataka*.

2. *Bahya-antar drishti*, which is outer and inner trataka combined.
3. *Adho trataka*, which is practised with the eyes half open and half closed.
4. *Antar drishti*, inner trataka, which is also known as *antaranga trataka*.
5. *Shoonya drishti*, which is gazing into the void.
6. *Nirantra drishti*, which is continuous gazing.

In trataka the different positions of the eyes have been studied and named. Open eyes are called *poornima drishti*, full vision. The full moon is also called poornima. Closed eyes are called *ama drishti*; *ama* relates to the word amavasya, and the no moon or dark moon is referred to as *amavasya*. Half-open eyes are called *pratipada drishti*. Poornima drishti is used in external trataka, ama drishti in inner trataka and pratipada drishti is made use of in adho trataka.

In outer trataka, or external gazing, the eyes remain open and focused on any steady object. This form of trataka can be practised by focusing the gaze on objects such as the flame of a candle, a dot, the rising sun and so on. By steadying the eyes in this manner the mind automatically becomes concentrated.

When outer and inner trataka are combined, one first gazes at an external point or object for some time, then closes the eyes and gazes at the after-image or inner reflection of the same object. Any object can be used for concentration. A luminous object, such as a candle flame, is often used by beginners as the brightness attracts the eyes and holds the gaze. It also imprints a clear image on the retina of the eyes which can be seen clearly when the eyes are closed.

This inner image becomes the object of concentration during antar trataka. If it is bright and clear enough, it holds the inner gaze so that one is aware of nothing else. This leads to concentration of the mental forces. The method of outer and inner trataka combined is useful for people who are not able to develop an inner image at will, without an external counterpart. Those who can create a steady, distinct inner image without the assistance of an outer object can practise inner trataka alone. In inner trataka the awareness is focused only on an internal image. Therefore, this practice is more difficult than outer trataka alone or outer and inner trataka combined. Inner trataka is most conducive to concentration as there is no external sensory contact, as there is with the other two forms. Inner trataka should be practised when one is able to create a clear inner image and when one's mind is reasonably tranquil and steady. If antar trataka is attempted when the inner image is vague, or there is no inner image, one either falls asleep or loses awareness in the usual patterns of thought play.

Shoonya drishti, gazing into the void should be practised after internal trataka has been mastered. *Shoonya* means the 'void' or 'formless state'. It is not chidakasha. In shoonya drishti there is no object of awareness. This form of trataka is done with the eyes open, gazing at nothingness. It takes a long time to come into this state. The eyes are open, but one is unable to see anything as the mind has become introverted. After some time the eyes become dim. They are half open and nothing can be seen. Nirantra drishti, continuous gazing, is looking at any point without blinking the eyes for hours together. It is what Ramana Maharshi used to practise, sitting for ten, eleven or twelve hours a day, without blinking his eyes.

How is bahir trataka practised?

Swami Niranjanananda: For external, or bahir trataka, an object or image which has a form is selected. Everything in the universe, the sun, moon, stars, trees, an idol or a photograph of the guru can be considered as symbols. One can practise bahir trataka making use of such an object, provided one's consciousness merges with it while gazing at it continuously.

Choose a symbol, bearing in mind that the symbol should not be changed. If it is changed, the after-image reflected on the screen of the mind becomes obsolete, and the practice needs to be started again from the beginning. Also, the full benefits of the practice will not be derived. If one selects a symbol and practises trataka on it daily, the after-image will start becoming clear. This will help later in the practice of inner trataka, and *chitta*, consciousness, will soon become steadily focused on that symbol.

Generally people are extroverted by nature, so for many people it is impossible to keep the eyes closed even for two minutes. Bahir trataka is useful here. Through bahir trataka the eyes are trained to be fixed and steady at one spot, so that the *chitta vrittis*, the patterns or dispositions of the mind, are changed and can easily be converted into introversion.

How is antar trataka practised?

Swami Niranjanananda: For inner, or antar trataka, the eyes are closed and the imaginative power of the mind is awakened. An image is fixed on the inner space of the mind, *chidakasha*, and then trataka is performed on it. For this an inner or mental symbol can be chosen. A *yantra*, geometric diagram, the sun or moon, one's own *ishta*, deity of choice, or the guru can be used as the symbol.

In the beginning, the practice of antaranga trataka is possible only after the practice of bahiranga trataka. With external trataka, the practice of concentrating chitta at one place is achieved and it helps an inner after-image to emerge. When the after-image appears clearly on the inner screen, chitta immediately becomes one pointed, as thoughts other than the after-image are obliterated. Once this is achieved, antar trataka is a highly effective practice to channel the energy on a definite path. Concentration and the state of meditation are attained with this type of trataka. People who can easily perceive the image of their symbol mentally can do antar trataka without first practising on an external object.

How is adho trataka practised?

Swami Niranjanananda: For adho trataka, practise with the eyes half open and half closed. Nasikagra drishti and shambhavi mudra are considered to be practices of adho trataka.

Why does the after-image seem to move around during antar trataka?

Swami Niranjanananda: It must be kept in mind that when antar trataka is practised, the symbol should remain still. When doing the practice, the symbol does not seem to remain in one place. There are physical and psychological reasons for this. First, the eyelids constantly flutter subtly; they are never steady. When the eyes are closed and one is trying to hold the inner gaze steady, fluttering eyelids disrupt the practice.

The second reason for unsteadiness is psychological. If the mind is restless, if it is not one-pointed, how can the after-image of the object be kept steady? If there is mental restlessness, the view does not remain stable for more than a few seconds. If trataka is practised when the mind is peaceful, the eyes will be steady. If trataka is practised immediately after activity, however, there will be inner excitement and the eyes will move more.

How can mudra and pranayama be integrated with trataka?

Swami Satyananda: As one becomes experienced at practising trataka, khechari mudra and ujjayi pranayama can be incorporated. In this technique, there is simultaneous awareness of the candle flame and the breath. Some imagination must also be used. While breathing in, one imagines that the breath is being drawn from the candle flame to the eyebrow centre and through to the back of the head. The awareness has to be split, so that it dwells on both the candle flame and the movement of the breath. There should also be awareness of the sound of the breath. When breathing out, one imagines that the breath flows from the back of the head, pierces the eyebrow centre and returns to the candle flame. The eyes should not flicker. This process continues: simultaneous awareness of the flame, the breath and its sound. Eventually, if one practises with sufficient intensity and awareness, it feels as if the air naturally and actually moves along the path between the flame and the back of the head.

The awareness of the breath can continue in this way when the eyes are closed and one is gazing at the after-image. Whilst breathing in, the breath is felt moving backwards from the flame in front of the closed eyes, to the back of the head. At the same time, one tries to draw the image backwards. Whilst breathing out, one imagines that the breath is being pushed forwards to the closed eyes, the image moving with the breath. Inhale and almost pull the image and breath backwards; exhale and push the image and the breath forwards. Kechari mudra and ujjayi are continued throughout. Awareness of the sound of ujjayi breathing is integrated with the movement of the breath from the eyebrow centre to the back of the head.

What can be done to help one feel the eyebrow centre during antar trataka?

Swami Satyananda: Throughout the practice of trataka the inner image has to be visualized and projected at the eyebrow centre. This is far easier if some kind of sensation is felt on the skin at that point. One method is to lick a finger just prior to commencing the practice and apply a dot at the eyebrow centre. This helps in the initial location of the correct position. However, the water soon evaporates. For this reason it is far better to apply a little menthol, camphor or tiger balm; these give a definite sensation at the eyebrow centre that lasts for the duration of the practice.

If one can easily feel the position of the eyebrow centre it is not necessary to use such methods.

How can trataka be practised during daily life?

Swami Sivananda: Trataka can be profitably done even when walking. While walking along the streets, do not look hither and thither. Gaze at the toes. Many people do not look at the face when they talk to others; their gaze is held at a particular place while they talk. No particular asana is required for this type of sadhana.

Does the way one gazes during trataka change as experience is gained?

Swami Satyananda: The sadhana of trataka is divided into two parts. The first is the elementary practice which is the process of gazing without flickering the eyelids. In this stage, trataka is practised on an object without thinking of its form, steadily and devoid of any mental changes. Trataka should be practised without any straining of the eyes; if the gazing is done in a natural state of mind, strain will be avoided. When the aspirant succeeds in practising trataka continuously for fifteen or twenty minutes without any feeling of fatigue for a few days, it is time to practise stage two.

The second part is practised with the eyes fixed as if they are trying to search for something: the process is as if one is carefully observing some objects or trying to find something small in a big thing. The eyeballs should be steady, there should be no strain, but at the same time the gazing should be with a purpose. Continuous practise leads to this experience.

The nature of the image has to be investigated as though looking for something. One must try to pierce through the exterior reality of the inner image by looking intently at the image and trying to probe its shape and nature. Gazing into the depths of the flame, perceiving as much detail as possible, one feels and sees the aura of the flame penetrating the mind. The collected rays of one's awareness have to probe the flame in an attempt to discover its deeper significance. What is the nature of the flame? What is the deeper essence behind what can be seen? This is continued for at least five to ten minutes or until the end of the practice. The longer the practice is maintained the better, especially if the inner image is exceptionally clear.

Although trataka is a simple practice, one has to be careful and alert when doing this sadhana, as one's vision and mental processes must be watched. If the mind is slightly active, the vision wanders away from the object. At the time of gazing the eyes should not be open too wide.

OBJECTS FOR TRATAKA

Does the hatha yoga tradition recommend different objects for trataka?

Swami Niranjanananda: The hatha yoga texts describe many forms of trataka of which the simplest and most commonly used is gazing at a candle flame. Trataka can also be practised by using various objects for concentration such as a yantra, chakra or mandala. Objects from nature can also be used, such as the moon, a star, a flower or a leaf.

How does one choose the object for trataka?

Swami Niranjanananda: The object should be something which naturally attracts one's attention and holds the gaze. Each practitioner must decide what is most suitable for himself. Commonly used objects include: candle flame, shivalingam, cross, nosetip, the symbol of *Om*, eyebrow centre, sky, another person's eyes, water, the symbol of yin yang, ishta devata, yantra or mandala, flower, one's own shadow, black dot, darkness, rising sun, reflection in a mirror, moon, crystal, star, shoonya, reflection of sun or moon in clear water.

Anything can be chosen as one's object, but once chosen, it should not be changed as this will decrease the effectiveness of the practice. If awareness is developed of one particular object and then it is suddenly changed, one must start from the beginning again to assimilate the new object. The mind has to mould itself around a particular object so that it is automatically drawn towards it. This takes time, so the object should be chosen carefully.

Can trataka be practised on ordinary objects?

Swami Satyananda: Take a glass full of white tea. Practise trataka on the decoction of that tea.

Trataka can be practised on a needle. Hang the needle on a plain coloured wall at eye level. There should be nothing else hanging on the wall as this will distract the attention during the practice. At the time of performing trataka, ensure that no other object is visible and that no other thought comes to mind.

Take any little article made of a bright metal, such as new vessels which shine when they are polished. Purchase any bright article from the bazaar; it may be of brass, copper, silver or gold; for example, an incense burner, or a small jug. It should not be more than two inches in height. Practise trataka on that bright object in half light.

Why is a candle flame usually recommended for trataka?

Swami Satyananda: The point of concentration is usually a symbol or object which activates the inner potential and can absorb the mind. The object most commonly used is a candle flame, as even after closing the eyes, the impression of the flame remains for some time and antaranga trataka can easily be practised. The purpose of focusing the eyes on an external object is to arouse the internal vision and to make that vision steady by stopping the eye movements.

There are other equally effective symbols or objects such as a crystal ball, a shivalingam, yantra, mandala, full moon, a star, the rising or setting sun (when it is an orange-red ball and not yellow), a chakra, the symbol of *Om*, or one's own shadow. These are the most effective, but trataka can also be done on a rose, a tree, a mountain, the sea, or lightning. In fact, when people worship a particular deity and gaze steadily at the form, that is also external trataka.

Of all the symbols and objects, however, the most suitable for general use is a candle flame. When a symbol, yantra or mandala is used, it leaves an impression in the mind and stimulates particular centres. For example, if one concentrates on Kali, that aspect of one's inner being is aroused if one is not beyond it. One may even manifest Kali and be terrified by her fearsome form. Therefore, a steady flame of light is most practical unless the guru says otherwise.

At a certain stage of concentration a point of light is seen in front of the closed eyes. This has to be developed and made steady, as initially it tends to waver or even disappear.

How is trataka practised on different forms of light?

Swami Sivananda: To practice trataka on a candle, place it in front and try to concentrate on the flame, without any eye movement. When the eyes become tired, close them and try to visualize the flame inside. This is done for half a minute and increased to five or ten minutes according to one's taste, temperament and capacity. One sees rishis and devatas, when deep concentration is entered into.

In a lying posture, concentrate on the moon. Whenever the mind runs, again and again bring it back to the image of the moon. This exercise is extremely beneficial for people who have an emotional temperament.

In the above manner, one can concentrate on any star that is singled out from the millions of stars shining above one's head.

Do visions occur when practising trataka on a flame?

Swami Sivananda: Place a ghee lamp or candle before you and gaze at the flame. Some astral entities give darshan through the flames.

What are the guidelines for gazing at the candle flame?

Swami Niranjanananda: With the eyes open, one looks at the brightest spot in the middle of the flame. It is essential to just gaze at the flame continuously, forgetting everything else. If the mind becomes unsteady it must be brought back and focused on the flame again. Different colours will be observed in the candle flame – in the middle the flame is a blackish area, which must be continuously looked at.

The main effort in trataka is to avoid twitching or blinking the eyelids. The eyes are kept open for as long as possible without creating any tension, from thirty to forty seconds up to two or three minutes. Before the eyes develop a burning sensation and tears start flowing, they are closed and kept closed while gazing at the after-image of the flame that appears in chidakasha. If the after-image cannot be seen at first, one should not worry, it will become clear with practice. In that case, the thought of the after-image should be kept clear at the back of the mind.

If a thought springs up, let it come; thoughts must be observed with a witnessing attitude. This is essential in the subtle practice of trataka. After each round the eyes are kept closed until their tiredness resolves and the after-image is no longer seen.

When the after-image becomes faint or disappears, and the eyes are relaxed, the eyes are opened and the practice is repeated. When intending to finish, the eyes are closed and when the after-image has faded, one continues watching chidakasha, the dark space in front of the closed eyes, for some time. Whatever appears there is watched while maintaining awareness of chidakasha. After a few minutes, the eyes are opened and the candle extinguished.

What is the method for practising trataka on a black dot?

Swami Satyananda: Take a big betel leaf. Prepare collyrium with the help of castor oil and make a black dot on the betel leaf. The dot should be of the size of a pea or a little smaller in size. Fix this leaf on cardboard. Alternatively, the black dot can be drawn on a white background and hung on a plain wall at eye level.

Behind, place a light, a lamp or a candle. Practise trataka on that dot in the morning and evening. Go on gazing at this dot continuously for five or ten minutes without moving the eyelids. Do this for six months, then consult the guru.

What size should objects such as a black dot, or symbols such as *Om* be for trataka?

Swami Niranjanananda: The size of the dot used for trataka differs for each individual. Each person must decide on the size of the dot, according to their eyesight. The important thing is not to strain the eyes. If two dots can be seen, it means either a smaller or a larger dot is needed. The same principle applies to concentration on the picture of one's guru, Shiva, Krishna, a yantra, mandala, *Om* or anything that is printed. This is to avoid adversely affecting the retina during the three minutes of external gazing. So, a dot of the proper size should be placed at the proper distance according to the eyesight capacity.

After gazing upon it for three minutes, the eyes are closed and awareness is of the inner vision. Internally, there will be a shadow with the same outline as the external object. If it is a cross, there will be a cross-like shadow. If it is an *Om* symbol, an *Om*-like shadow will appear. If it is a crescent moon, a crescent shadow will appear. If it is a human figure, a human shadow will be there. This shadow is concentrated on in the same manner as in trataka on the candle flame. The effect on the retina is different, as one is not seeing a luminous object. When gazing at the shadow of the black dot it may be black, blue, grey, or any colour. It will disappear, reappear, disappear, etc. When it can no longer be seen, one starts a new round.

How is trataka practised on a flower?

Swami Niranjanananda: Any flower may be used for this practice. It is best if the colour is deep and strong. If it is a red rose, trataka is performed in a bright place. If the flower is white, yellow or pink, a black or dark green cloth about two feet wide and three feet long is needed. The flower is pinned to the centre of the cloth. Trataka should then be practised in a dimly lit place.

How is trataka performed on a picture of one's ishta devata?

Swami Sivananda: A picture of one's *ishta devata*, personal deity, is placed in front of the eyes. Suppose one is doing trataka on Lord Vishnu: the mind is first fixed on the feet of Lord Vishnu, then on the lotus under the legs. Move the gaze

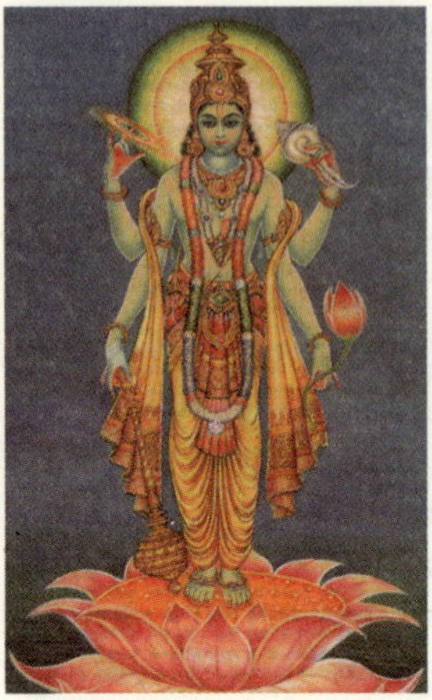

Vishnu

around the yellow silken cloth, the *pitambara*, then to the golden *hara*, the gem on the breast, then the earring, the face, the crown on the head, the bracelets on the arm, the disc in the right upper hand, the conch in the left upper hand, then the *gada*, mace, in the left lower hand. This is the order. Then bring the gaze down to the feet and start again, moving towards the upper parts. In this way, practise again and again. Whenever the mind runs away, fix it, just as Lord Krishna says in the *Bhagavada Gita* (6:26):

> *Yato yato nischarati manaschanchalamasthiram;*
> *Tatastato niyamyaitad aatmanyeva vasam nayet.*
>
> From whatever cause the restless, unsteady mind wanders away, from that let him restrain it and bring it under the control of the Self alone.

In the picture of Vishnu, the conch represents *Om* or shabdha Brahman. The disc is the destroyer of the evil vrittis or vasanas, the mace represents the emblem of sovereignty, the lotus at his feet represents the world or universe.

How is trataka practised on one's chosen deity?

Swami Satyananda: To practise trataka on one's chosen deity, a small photograph of the deity is used. Then, in the centre of a sheet of black paper the size of a book, a circle two inches in diameter is cut. The photo is fixed behind the paper in such a manner that only the face of the deity can be seen through that hole. The picture is placed at eye level, approximately one arm's length from the eyes.

Practise this form of trataka during the day. The photo should be directly in front of the eyes, one and a half inches away. One should not see anything except that which is within the circle, and should try not to look at anything else.

How is trataka performed on a Shivalinga?

Swami Satyananda: To perform trataka on the Shivalinga it must be worshipped daily with great devotion. The Shivalinga must be of black stone. During the worship, one concentrates on the water as it is poured on the linga. A sandalwood mark is then made on it and the eyes are steadied on that mark. One can also try to concentrate on that entire black linga.

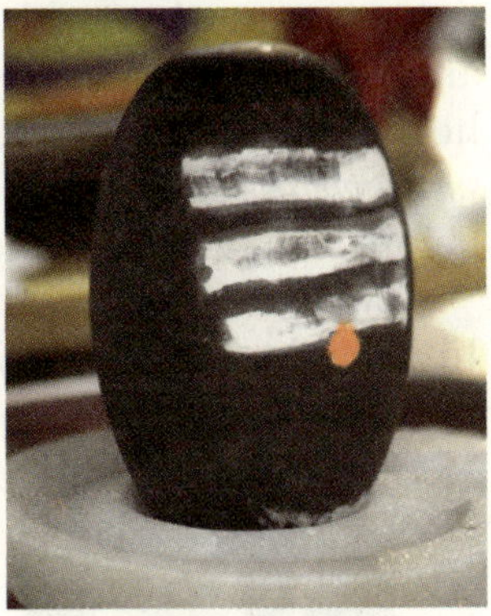
Black lingam

What is the significance of practising trataka on a jyotirlingam?

Swami Niranjanananda: The best form of trataka is gazing on the jyotirlingam. This is a luminous, oval-shaped crystal. Natural crystals of this shape are found in the Narmada River in India, and this is the traditional source of the jyotirlingam. If the jyotirlingam is placed under a flow of water at any time of day, it produces different shades of colours, visions and outlines, where snakes, elephants, jungles, rivers, landscapes and worlds being born and destroyed may be seen. There are twelve places in India where jyotirlingams have been established: Somnatheshwar, Mallikarjuna, Mahakaleshwar, Omkareshwar, Kedareshwar, Bheemashankar, Vishweshwar, Tryambakeshwar, Vaidyanatheshwar, Nageshwar, Grishneshwar and Rameshwar. These are the jyotirlingams on which trataka is practised.

Everything which exists in the physical universe is drawn from the basis of an inner reality. The great seers saw the lingam inside and that vision gave rise to an outer symbol. In the Upanishads it is said that trataka on an external shivalingam is synonymous to concentration on the internal astral body. The oval shape, which is seen outside, is the same shape seen within oneself as the astral body.

By practising trataka on the jyotirlingam, the aspirant comes face to face with himself and learns the secret of birth and death. He is able to fulfil his spiritual ambitions. Finally, he sees the eternal life inside himself. This jyotirlingam is *swayambhu*, self-created, self-born. Nobody created it. It existed before birth, as the subtle body existed before the physical body.

This jyotirlingam manifests differently on different planes. In the physical world it is seen in temples. On the higher planes of consciousness it is seen in the form of light. In order to worship this jyotirlingam there is no need to use prayer, mantra or flower offerings. One simply has to sit down before the lingam, place a bilwa leaf in front of it, pour water over it and gaze into it, trying to assimilate its physical form within. Nothing else is necessary. It does not matter if one is a believer or not. It is a universal symbol.

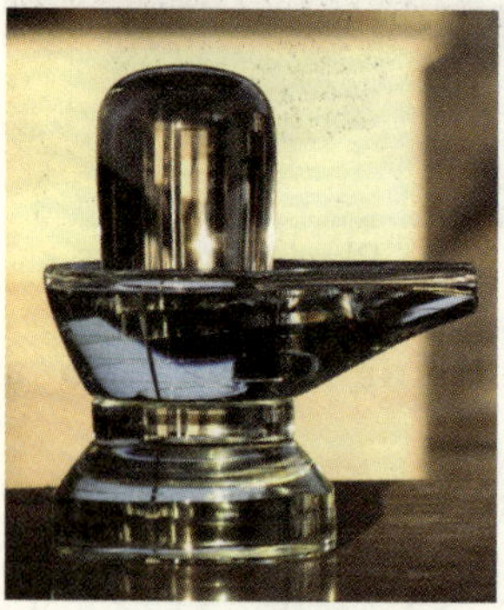
Crystal lingam

Can trataka be practised on a crystal ball?

Swami Satyananda: Trataka can be practised on a big or small crystal ball. Crystal balls are of two types, those which are transparent and those which are not transparent.

How is trataka practised on crystal?

Swami Niranjanananda: When crystal is used as an object for concentration one must practise in dim light, in a room which is neither too bright nor too dark. A black cloth is spread on a table. Then a stand is placed on the table and the crystal on the stand. One assumes a meditation posture, closes the eyes and establishes body stillness, then the eyes are opened and the gaze is directed into the crystal. The consciousness and the vision must penetrate the centre of the crystal. Nothing will be seen. Here trataka on an external object and on shoonya are combined. When one gazes into the crystal for a long time, the mind goes blank and visions begin to come, even while the eyes are open.

Usually the period fixed for gazing upon an external object is from three to five minutes. However, there is an exception to the rule in this practice. In crystal gazing one can concentrate for ten minutes, but tears should not fall and the eyes should not be strained. One should continue gazing into the crystal for as long as possible without blinking the eyes. The eye muscles should remain absolutely relaxed. The eyelids should not flicker. The moment strain is felt, the eyes should be closed and rested. There is no need to think of the crystal when the eyes are closed. Concentration comes quickly while focusing on crystal.

This practice develops telepathy, for crystal has the property of attracting sound waves. Radios also contain crystals which attract sound waves, but these are synthetic crystals. The properties of real crystals are more subtle and powerful.

How is trataka practised on the sky?

Swami Niranjanananda: When practising trataka on the sky, sit outside in an open place or on a terrace where there is nothing obstructing the view. Sitting in any comfortable meditation posture, kaya sthairyam is practised for some time, until the body becomes still and quiet. The awareness is then brought to chidakasha, where any thoughts or images are watched. Gradually the mental activity lessens and the mind becomes quiet. When this state occurs, the eyes are opened and one gazes steadily at the blue sky. The eyes should not blink or flicker in any way. Slowly one lets the awareness of the surroundings slip away, and becomes aware only of the vast blue space of the sky; it seems that there is nothing else but the sky. As one gazes, it feels as if the sky is coming closer and closer; one feels the sky moving in all directions and allows oneself to be enveloped within the vastness of the sky. This awareness is intensified, becoming deeper and more intense, until one has the experience of becoming part of the sky, as if there is no difference between oneself and the sky. One becomes the sky, experiencing the endless space; awareness is of experiencing this space, this sky. To end the practice the eyes are closed and one lets go of the awareness of the sky and externalizes the mind.

What happens when trataka is practised on the moon or stars?

Swami Sivananda: Lie down on an open terrace and gaze at a particular bright star or the full moon. After some time, different colours of lights are seen. Some time later, only one colour is seen throughout, and all other stars disappear. When gazing at the moon, only a bright moon on a black background is seen. At times a huge mass of light will be seen all around one's self. When gazing becomes more intense, two or three moons of the same size can be seen, and at times no moon at all can be seen, even though one's eyes may be wide open.

How does one practise trataka on the sun and moon?

Swami Niranjanananda: When practising trataka on the sun or moon one must never gaze directly at them. The sun's rays can damage the retina and cause cataracts in the eyes. Practising trataka directly on the moon can create mental imbalance and a person can become moonstruck. Anyone suffering from any kind of mental disturbances or depression should not do this practice. Trataka on the sun and moon are powerful practices as they have a direct effect on the ida and pingala energies in the body and mind, so care should be taken.

The sun increases the flow of energy in the pingala nadi, increasing dynamism, while the moon affects ida nadi, increasing the mental force. Those wishing to increase their dynamic, vital powers should do trataka on the rising or setting sun. Those wishing to delve into and uncover their mental potential should practise trataka on the rising or setting moon.

When doing trataka on the sun or moon a pea-sized circular hole should be cut in the centre of a large square of dark-coloured cloth. This cloth should be attached to a window facing the sun or moon or to a separate frame that can be used outside. Trataka should then be done by gazing at the sun or moon through this hole.

The practice is done in the same way as when using a candle flame, gazing both at the external image and the internal image. One should try to be aware of the finer and more subtle effects the sun or moon have upon the prana, the body and mind, for example, any changes in the flow of energy and any mood changes. As the practice continues, the awareness is allowed to become deeper and more subtle.

What is the method for practising trataka on darkness?

Swami Satyananda: Sit alone in the dark and practise trataka on the darkness. The eyes should be fully open. Continue to see the darkness without any light. Sit there daily and practise it steadily and firmly.

What happens when one practises trataka on darkness?

Swami Niranjanananda: This practice is similar to practising trataka on the sky. Trataka on darkness should be practised where there is complete darkness, where nothing can be seen, not even one's own hand. One sits with eyes open, gazing into the darkness. The gaze must be held steady and still. One keeps looking into that darkness for as long as possible without causing strain to the eyes. If thoughts or emotions come, let them, but the attention is fixed on the darkness. One tries to penetrate the darkness. After some time the darkness vanishes and visions start floating.

According to some psychologists who have made experiments on this particular form of trataka, it is one of those practices by which the subconscious mind and behaviour, the suppressed feelings, phobias and fears, come up in the form of visions and float in that darkness. One must not become caught up and involved in these images and visions; one should be aware of them but not be disturbed by them.

As this is such a powerful practice it is not recommended for those people who have an impure, restless or abnormal mind. When the subconscious mind begins to manifest, such people will not be able to understand what is happening and their fears will be increased. Therefore, trataka on darkness should only be practised by those who have sufficient mental control and detachment, and who have been leading a pure, disciplined inner life. In that state they will see the higher astral plane.

How is trataka practised on one's own eye?

Swami Sivananda: Look at a mirror and gaze at the pupil of the eye.

Can antar trataka be practised on the chakras?

Swami Sivananda: Advanced students can do trataka on the chakras. Mooladhara, anahata, ajna and sahasrara are the important centres for trataka.

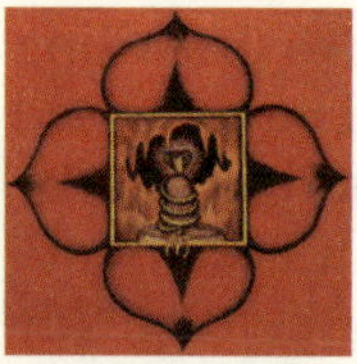

Mooladhara

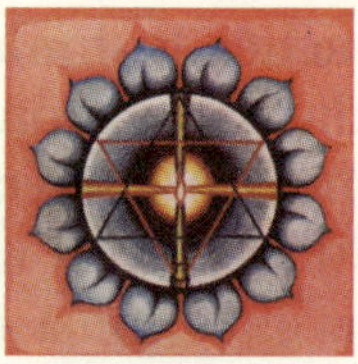

Anahata

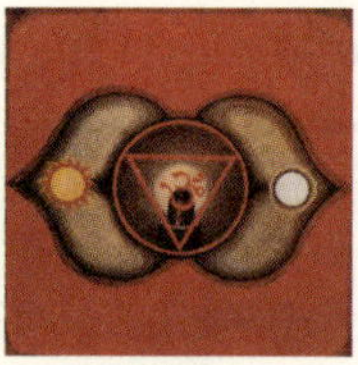

Ajna

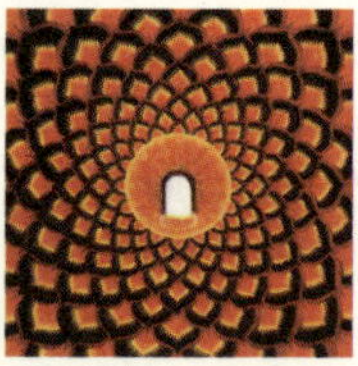

Sahasrara

How is trataka performed on havan?

Swami Niranjanananda: When performing havan, scented items are put into the sacrificial fire. When the fire is burning steadily, the gaze is focused and held steadily on the centre of the fire. The eyes must not move in any way. One continues looking deeply into the fire, letting go of the external surroundings, letting any thoughts that come just pass by. With one's full attention concentrated on the fire, it feels as if one is moving closer to the fire. The feeling is that there is nothing but the fire; the fire is experienced as if it were part of oneself. One tries to understand the real nature of the fire and to be aware of the divine within the fire, without intellectualizing or trying too hard. One should just be open to the fire and try to see the fire as it really is. The awareness goes deeper and deeper into the fire, and the steady concentrated gaze continues as long as there is no strain or discomfort. Then the eyes are closed, and in a state of silence the awareness goes inside, so that the experience is of whatever is happening within. Finally the awareness is returned to the physical body and the mind is fully externalized.

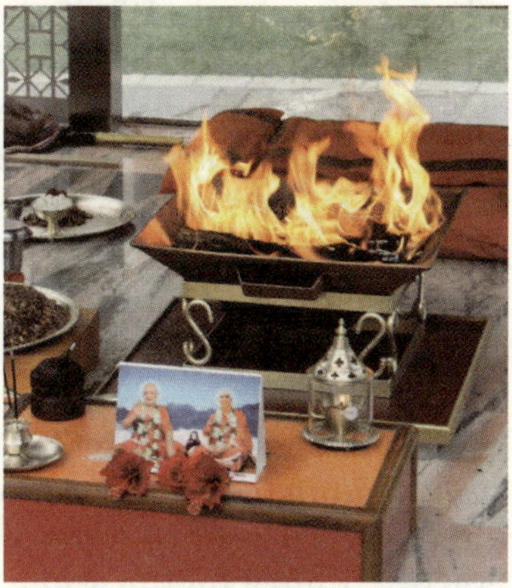
Havan

Can trataka be practised on a moving scene, for example, while travelling?

Swami Niranjanananda: Trataka can be done while travelling by train or car. One needs to sit beside an open window and relax the whole body. The body and mind should be settled by practising awareness of body and breath, so that other sounds, of other passengers or the train itself, fade into the background.

Then, with the eyes open, one gazes at the distant scene. At first this may be difficult as the eyes automatically follow the moving scenery. It takes a few moments until the eyes are able to settle on one point. They are then held steady, without straining. The eyelids should not flicker and the eyeballs should not move even though the scene is constantly changing. The eyes are kept focused on the middle of the scene. There should be no thoughts or emotions as one gazes at the distant scene. The mind should be completely steady and devoid of all emotions. There is awareness of the continuously changing scenes but without judging them or becoming involved in them.

Concentration is completely on the centre of the distant scene, where the eyes are kept steady and focused. If the eyes become tired they can be closed for a few moments and relaxed completely. While the eyes are closed, the awareness is brought to the eyebrow centre. One must not be distracted by any surrounding sounds and movements. The awareness must be continually brought back to the practice. When the eyes feel rested, they are again opened and the gaze is fixed on the distant scene. The practice continues in this way. When the practice is finished, the eyes are closed and allowed to completely relax.

How can trataka be practised on a river?

Swami Satyananda: Sit down on a river bank or raised ground where the current of water can be seen for a long distance. Practise trataka on the water. The eye should remain steadily fixed on one spot. It should not move along the waves.

How is trataka practised on a current of water?

Swami Niranjanananda: To practise trataka on moving water, one sits on a river bank or raised ground near the river. The flow of water should be visible for a long distance. It is essential to sit in a steady comfortable posture so that the body will not move in any way during the practice. One must always remain fully alert when practising trataka on water. The gaze is fixed on one point and should remain steady, with awareness of the continuous flowing movement of the water, but without moving along the ripples. If this happens, the gaze is gently brought back to the central point of concentration. There should be complete one-pointed awareness, with continuous gazing at the current of water for as long as possible without straining the eyes. Then the eyes are closed and allowed to relax completely. The awareness is brought to the eyebrow centre, and one becomes aware of the effects of the practice on different levels, from the physical to the more subtle.

How is trataka practised on a yantra?

Swami Niranjanananda: A suitable yantra is selected, for example, Sri Yantra. The yantra is placed on a stand so that it is upright and at eye level. The entire diagram should be seen clearly without any strain to the eyes. The yantra should be drawn in black and white or on a copper plate in the beginning. Later on coloured yantras may be drawn.

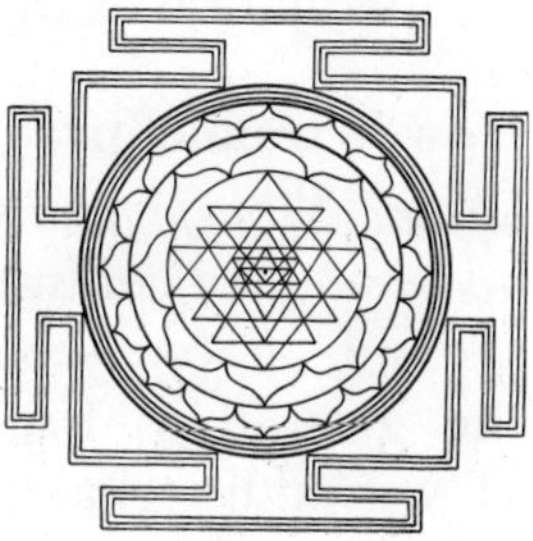

Sri Yantra

How is trataka practised on a three-dimensional form?

Swami Niranjanananda: Whenever trataka is practised on objects with a three dimensional form, one must be particularly aware of the dimensions. Here it is not only awareness of the object, but awareness of the dimensions which is important.

When doing this practice one should choose a pleasant object and concentrate on that object. One may choose a dog, for example. The mind should not be totally absorbed in the dog, but one should try to relate to relevant objects and ideas which are connected with the dog. The dog remains the central theme. The mind must not be allowed to wander off onto a completely irrelevant line of thought. One must think of the shape of the dog, think of the different types of dogs. The mind must be brought back to the central object, the dog. Think of the food the dog eats. Think of the close relationship that exists between dog and man. Return to the central object. Continue in this way, bringing in as many related topics as possible. One must not allow the mind to think of anything that is unrelated.

Different objects can be chosen when the exploration of one object has been exhausted. This is an excellent way of developing the power to control ideas and thoughts at will. It is an invaluable method of training the mind to follow a fixed path of association instead of jumping from one subject to a totally unrelated topic. It is useful for training the mind for meditation as well as everyday activity.

How is trataka practised on one's shadow?

Swami Niranjanananda: This practice is known as *chhaya upasana*, 'concentration on one's shadow'. Standing with the sun at one's back, one gazes at the shadow cast on the ground in front. The gaze is focused at the point of vishuddhi chakra on the shadow. There is no special indication there: this point has to be created mentally. One continues gazing steadily at vishuddhi on the shadow for five minutes or for as long as one can. When it is not possible to gaze at the shadow for even one second more, one stops and looks directly up into the sky. While gazing upward, a great shadow cast over the background of the sky will be perceived. It will be silver in colour and somewhat hazy. One goes on gazing at the shadow until it disappears, then tries to reassemble it as one does in other trataka practices when the eyes are closed. It is difficult to gather it again in the beginning, but it may be possible to do it once or twice. Then the eyes are closed and relaxed completely. When they are rested one can again resume gazing on the shadow at the point of vishuddhi. After a few minutes, one looks up quickly without any delay and gazes steadily into the sky. This is continued until the shadow in the sky takes on the form of one's own shadow.

How is trataka practised on one's own reflection?

Swami Niranjanananda: Trataka can be practised on one's own reflection in a mirror or in a still body of water, such as a pond or lake. The best time to practise this is when the sun is high in the sky, not at night or on a cloudy or rainy day. If it is dark outside, there should be sufficient light in the room so that the eyes are not strained. When trataka is practised on one's own reflection, it must always be remembered that whatever is seen is a projection or manifestation of one's own self. Nothing comes from outside. While practising this form of trataka, if any psychic apparitions are experienced, it is better to leave the practice.

GUIDELINES FOR PRACTICE

What are the general guidelines for practising trataka?

Swami Satyananda: The practice of trataka on any object can be performed during the day or night. In this practice, one must take into account the object, the place and the time. At the time of practising, the eyeballs should remain steady and the eyelids should not flicker; no other object should be seen, and the mind should not wander hither and thither, but should be merged in the observation of that object.

What state of mind should be adopted when practising trataka?

Swami Satyananda: Trataka is not just looking intently at an object, it is looking at the object with awareness and mindfulness, as one does while looking in a mirror. Complaints are received that sometimes trataka injures the eyes, but this is due to the sadhaka overstraining the eyes. If one gazes upon the object as one gazes into a mirror at one's own reflection, with simple awareness and mindfulness, trataka will help immensely. Also, one should not enter into analysis of the object of trataka during the practice. The proper way to practise is to look steadily at the object, with awareness and mindfulness.

What obstacles does the sadhaka face when practising trataka?

Swami Satyananda: Certain difficulties are encountered during trataka sadhana. Those who are not used to sitting in one posture for a long time, may have problems sitting comfortably and still. In the beginning, it is difficult to keep the eyes steady, as naturally, the eyelids tend to drop. It is hard to stop this, even with effort made over a long time. This creates an additional problem, as when the eyelides drop, it is difficult to gaze steadily and continuously on one central point.

Other difficulties are that the eyes get watery, and continuous gazing at an object may make it appear double, which is to be avoided. Sometimes the black spot appears white and vice versa, and most difficult of all, the sadhaka is often overcome by uncontrollable sleep during the practice of trataka.

A sadhaka has to overcome these obstacles, and it is not difficult to do so if one is alert and firmly fixed in one's ideal. For people of firm determination, difficulty is surmountable. The practice should be increased gradually and slowly. A concentrated mind is a great help to an aspirant. Everything becomes easy to one who practises with devotion, firmness and honesty.

What should be done if trataka causes mental disturbance?

Swami Satyananda: Everyone has accumulated complexes and problems stored in the mind. The aim of yoga is to clean out the mind of this accumulated dross. Trataka is an excellent method in this respect for it helps one to become aware of one's problems. However, it is possible for the problems to manifest too rapidly, with possible mental upsets. If this occurs, the practice should be stopped and expert advice sought.

Can trataka lead to frightening visions?

Swami Satyananda: There is a way, a method and a definite process of practising trataka. Trataka can bring about the awakening of one's monstrous psychic being. Therefore, even when practising trataka for the eyes or for curing insomnia, it should be done correctly so that the wrong psychic explosions do not develop.

Some people practise trataka and they see hell, monsters, ghosts, and such horrible things, so they stop the practice. They thought that perhaps these things really had come down, but actually it was all an expression of what was suppressed in them. Therefore, when trataka is practised there is a system according to what is being looked at, and the duration of the practice should not be too long.

If trataka is practised too intensely, or on the wrong object, can it cause mental disorientation?

Swami Niranjanananda: It has been observed that prisoners who remain in a cell all day sometimes lie on their bed continually, looking only at the ceiling or a lighted bulb. This is a form of trataka, and they often hallucinate and cannot tolerate or handle the experiences it brings up. An internal change takes place in which they feel their own identity is coming to an end, they are removed from the outside world and from external experiences. To lose one's self-identity is a person's greatest insecurity. Losing their fortune or having their house burn down will cause some suffering, but it will be much less than that caused by the loss of self-identity. This is a big blow, which destroys the entire mental structure.

In this way, one sometimes almost unconsciously adopts something and concentrates the gaze on it. In yoga, however, one should take care that the symbolic object is the correct one, and to practise only under guidance. In *Gheranda Samhita,* Sage Gheranda recommends 'a subtle object' in his explanation; a simple candle flame is often used.

What precautions should be taken when practising trataka?

Swami Niranjanananda: Do not practise trataka on a flame that is not steady. People with visual problems should ensure that the symbol is positioned so that a double image is not seen, and should seek expert guidance if this is not possible. Generally speaking, trataka should not be practised wearing spectacles.

Although the texts specifically mention tears, notice that the wording indicates practising until the threshold of this experience. The point of the practice is not to make tears roll down the face, but simply to practise as long as one can without this happening.

People with glaucoma should not practise trataka. Epileptics should not practise trataka on a candle flame. Trataka should not be practised on the sun.

For how long should trataka be practised?

Swami Sivananda: Do trataka for two minutes to start with, then cautiously increase the period. Do not be impatient; gradual steady practice is required. Even gazing at a spot for a full three hours counts for nothing if the mind is wandering. The mind must also be on the spot: only then does one advance in this practice and attain many psychic powers.

However, those who cannot gaze steadily in spite of several attempts need not worry; they should close their eyes and gaze at an imaginary spot in the space between the two eyebrows.

Those who have weak eye capillaries should do trataka after closing their eyes – they can focus on any imaginary spot within. Similarly, when tired, close the eyes and keep the mind on the object of trataka. Do not tax the eyes by too much practice.

How much time should be spent on the outer and inner stages of trataka?

Swami Satyananda: The longer one is able to practise the internal stage of the practice the better. In other words, if a clear inner image can easily be retained, the external stage can be reduced or even eliminated. Of course, if a clear after-image cannot be seen, the duration of the external stage should be increased.

During the external stage, one should continue to gaze at the flame for as long as possible without flickering the eyes.

Beginners should aim at about two or three minutes. With practice, the time can be increased up to five or ten minutes at one stretch.

Beginners who cannot see an image should try to create or discern an image for a minute or so and then open their eyes. Advanced practitioners may find that they can see an image almost indefinitely. If that is so, inner trataka can be practised throughout, or for as long as the image can be seen. The aim is to increase the duration of inner trataka and eventually reduce the period assigned to outer trataka, as generally inner trataka is far more conducive to meditation and awareness of the deeper layers of the mind.

To gain noticeable benefits try to practise for at least fifteen minutes every day; more if possible. Trataka can be practised at any time, though early in the morning and late at night are ideal. If possible practise at both these times. Practice should be done at a time when there will be no outer disturbances.

The number of rounds or repetitions depends entirely on the ability to retain the inner image. Those who are more proficient may only need to do one round, for they will be able to hold the inner image throughout the duration of the practice. Beginners, on the other hand, will need to do a number of repetitions according to their proficiency and the duration of the practice.

When and for what duration should trataka be practised?

Swami Niranjanananda: Trataka can be done at any time, but it is more effective when practised on an empty stomach. The most suitable time is between four and six in the morning. If the aim is to delve deeper into the mind, trataka should be practised late at night before going to bed and before japa or meditation. The ideal times for practising are early morning or at night.

Trataka is a heat producing practice, so it should be done after bathing, when one feels fresh. If surya namaskara is practised before trataka, the body is heated, causing discomfort during trataka; the body should be kept cool before practising trataka. If one practices meditation after doing trataka, the body will again become cool and refreshed.

It is said that if the object of concentration is physical in nature, such as a flame, trataka should not be practised for more than five minutes. The duration depends on the individual, however, it is essential to obtain directions from an experienced guide if intending to practise for longer. Five minutes of practice is sufficient to remove some types of eye defects.

What posture is best for trataka?

Swami Niranjanananda: Trataka must be practised in the steadiest possible posture. Although it can be done sitting in a chair or in sukhasana, it is far better to practise it in siddhasana or padmasana.

One can sit in any meditative asana in which the body can be kept steady. The back and neck should be in a straight line. The candle should be placed on a stand at eye level, about an arm's length away from the eyes, so that the back and head can be kept straight when gazing at it.

The whole body must become like a statue. It is essential to be aware of the state of the body. Physical stability is important, as there should be no movement in the body to disturb the concentration. Once the practice begins there should be absolutely no movement of the body.

Do the various objects require different amounts of light?

Swami Niranjanananda: When using a black dot or any other object, there should be good light. Crystal gazing is done in dim light. When using a candle flame, there should be no other light. Trataka on a candle flame must be practised in a room without a fan, where there is no breeze. The candle flame should not flicker. The candle should be placed on a firm stand at eye level, about an arm's length away.

How important is it to keep the eyes absolutely still?

Swami Niranjanananda: In both the external and internal forms of trataka the eyes should not blink or move in any way. Stillness of the eyeballs and eyelids is essential in order to attain clarity of the inner image. If the eyes feel at all strained, imagine breathing through the eyebrow centre to and from ajna chakra. If they still feel strained, close them. When the eyes are closed, gaze at the after-image and continue the same awareness of the breath, breathing to and from the image through the eyebrow centre. The mind should be focused on the object or image and nothing else. If the mind wanders or starts to think about other things, bring it back to the object of concentration.

Can trataka be done by those with defective vision?

Swami Niranjanananda: Trataka on any object is better practised without eyeglasses or contact lenses. If one has defective vision, the object must be positioned so that there is no double vision and the object is not blurred.

How can trataka be practised on the rising sun?

Swami Niranjanananda: If trataka is practised on the rising sun, never look at the sun directly. This is harmful to the eyes and may cause cataracts. Gaze upon the sun's reflection on clear water. When the reflection is disturbed by heavy wind or storm, this form of trataka should not be practised.

What should one do when thoughts crowd the mind during trataka?

Swami Niranjanananda: In the yogic practice of trataka one meditates on a flame or some other symbolic object. Often when the eyes are focused on the flame, many thoughts spring up. They should be allowed to come, observe them as a witness. It is important to remember the aim or objective. Trying to suppress thoughts increases mental tension. So if thoughts come, let them come. Keep the attitude of a witness and the thoughts will go of their own accord. This attitude is described in *Hatharatnavali* (1:52):

Atha Traataka
Nireekshya nishchaladrishaa sookshmalakshyam samaahitah.
Ashrusampaataparyantamaachaaryaistrotakam smritam.

Now trataka: Well composed and keeping the sight steady, one should stare at a small object until tears come out. This is called trataka by the teachers.

Is there any particular way to breathe during the practice of trataka?
Swami Satyananda: During the practice of trataka the breathing must be slow, rhythmic and deep. This brings steadiness to the breathing process.

Does it matter if there is background noise while practising trataka?
Swami Niranjanananda: Trataka should be done in absolute silence.

HEALTH BENEFITS

Why should one practise trataka?
Swami Sivananda: Trataka improves eyesight. Diseases of the eyes are removed. Many have thrown away their spectacles after some practice of trataka. It develops the power of concentration to a great degree. Trataka practice gives tremendous power, removes a host of eye troubles, and bestows *divya drishti*, divine vision.

Do the various objects used in trataka have different effects?
Swami Satyananda: There are various branches of trataka: one can practise trataka on water, fire, earth, sky, ether, air, a dot, light, chidakasha or on any steady object. Each has its own cluster of significant attributes. Certain practices improve

the eyesight, while others are helpful in removing certain cerebral congestions and reviving memory. It depends upon one's requirement, whether a shining substance or a dark object is needed. Trataka on a *sphatik*, crystal, shivalinga is considered the best of all forms of trataka.

What are the physiological benefits of trataka?

Swami Niranjanananda: Physiologically trataka relieves eye ailments such as eyestrain and headache, myopia, astigmatism and even early stages of cataract. It can help to remove nervous tics or uncontrolled nervous activity such as one eye blinking very fast. The eyes become clear and bright, able to see the reality beyond appearances. Trataka benefits not only the eyes, but a whole range of physiological and mental functions. It is therapeutic for depression, insomnia, allergy, anxiety and postural problems. In *Hatharatnavali* (1:53) the benefits are given:

> *Sphotanam netrarogaanaam tantraadeenaam kavaatakam.*
> *Prayatnaattrotanam gopyam yathaaratnam supetakam.*
>
> Trataka, which clears eye diseases and prevents sloth should be valued and kept secret with the same effort as one keeps a casket of precious stones.

How effective is trataka at reducing anxiety?

Swami Niranjanananda: In normal conditions the concentration practice of trataka, fixing the gaze in the middle of a candle flame, helps to improve concentration and one-pointed awareness. In extreme conditions, such as soldiers in remote and dangerous locations, research has shown that trataka helps to stop dissipation of the emotions and thoughts, and to reduce the level of fear, insecurity and anxiety.

How can yoga help insomnia?

Swami Satyananda: For insomnia, first practice trataka, then yoga nidra. These practices will relieve insomnia, but there is something else one has to do. Why does one have insomnia? Because one thinks and thinks and thinks.

What effect does trataka have on sleep and melatonin?

Swami Niranjanananda: The sixth shatkarma is trataka, which is one of the important practices of pratyahara. If trataka is practised at night before going to bed, when one lies down, the mind is absolutely quiet, there is no *vikshepa* of mind, there is no confusion or movement of mind. Trataka is a most effective technique to focus the mind, clearing it of confusion, conflict, stress and tension. The brain has a large visual centre. When the vision is confined to observing a flame only, and the eyes are not moving around grasping objects and seeing images, the brain is not processing them, so at that time there is cerebral relaxation. The cerebral relaxation combined with mental harmony and the state of concentration changes the entire quality of sleep, consciousness and mind.

Australian research has shown that trataka practised at night on a candle flame stimulates the production of melatonin. Melatonin is a hormone produced by the pineal gland in the head. The pineal gland is inactive during the day, but with the coming of darkness it wakes up and secretes melatonin. Melatonin is an important hormone which regulates the body clock: it is only produced at night, in darkness, and it causes one to feel sleepy, ready for bed. Melatonin also helps regulate the female reproductive cycle and has powerful antioxidant effects, meaning it enhances the immune system. With the coming of dawn, melatonin levels subside, and one is ready to wake and start the day.

Research has shown that if trataka is practised at night on a flame, for only one or two minutes, the melatonin production increases. It must be practised in darkness, and after this brief practice, one must go straight to bed, without turning on the light. Bright light stops the effect. The quality of sleep is totally different when trataka is practised at night.

Along with practising trataka, a regulated lifestyle is a must. Irregular sleep and waking times, dietary indiscretions, high stress levels, indulgence in sensory pleasures and an unbalanced attitude towards life, all put off the desired effects.

Trataka can also have the opposite effect: if it is practised for too long, people often find that they can't sleep. When trataka is practised, the mind relaxes, as the state of concentration stops the mind from distracting itself and going in hundreds of directions, giving birth to different kinds of thoughts. When the mind is concentrated, the thoughts automatically align themselves and there is no dissipation or distraction. This is an alert state, not a drowsy state. The eyes are the *jnanendriya*, the sense organ, of manipura chakra, therefore when trataka is practised for some time, it has an effect on manipura, making one feel energetic. If trataka is practised for half an hour, after that there will be no sleep, no matter how tired or exhausted one was before.

Furthermore, if trataka is practised on an object other than a candle flame, there must be light, and in light, the melatonin effect cannot occur. Sleep is a necessity for the maintenance of health, but if one wants to overcome sleep, trataka can be an effective technique. Even if one is able to sleep, the quality of sleep is different; it is deep, relaxing and short.

It should be remembered that the state of relaxation arising from trataka is important for another reason: once there is sufficient relaxation, one acquires concentration, and the attitudes change. The attitude changes with the relaxation of mind and it is this change in attitude, it is this relaxation of mind, which makes one's life happier and healthier. In yoga one aspires to live gracefully: that grace is an outcome of a harmonious and balanced perception of life.

SUBTLE EFFECTS

What is the main purpose for practising trataka?

Swami Sivananda: Trataka, the practice of steady gazing at a particular point or object without blinking, is mainly intended for developing the powers of concentration and mental focus. When one gazes at a particular point or picture, it is trataka. This is useful for everyone.

How can trataka help one control the senses?

Swami Sivananda: Control the ears by hearing the glories, the lilas and kirtans of the Lord, and by hearing the anahata sounds with the practice of yoni mudra.

Control the sense of touch by practice of brahmacharya, sleeping on a coarse mat, using a coarse blanket, wearing a coarse shirt and coarse clothes.

Practise trataka daily to control the wandering eyes. Feel that every form is the form of the Lord. Put a stamp of the picture of the Lord on every mental form. Do trataka on your ishta devata and visualize the picture with closed eyes.

Give up those articles which the mind likes best for a week or a month. Give up salt on Sundays. Take sugarless milk. Abandon pickles and chutney. Do not ask for extra salt, or sugar for tea or milk. Take simple, bland food. Fast on ekadashi, amavasya, poornima, janmashtami, Shivaratri, and dussehra.

What mental and psychic faculties are developed by practising trataka?

Swami Sivananda: With the practice of trataka willpower is developed. Vikshepa is destroyed. The mind is steadied. Clairvoyance, thought reading, psychic cure and other siddhis are easily obtained.

What are the effects of trataka on the brain?

Swami Satyananda: Trataka is an important practice and a direct method of influencing the brain. The eye is actually an extension of the brain and the optic nerve is one of the twelve cranial nerves that emerge from the brain, not the spinal cord, so therefore, when the optic system is engaged, the brain is influenced.

The yogis discovered that making the eyes steady by gazing at a point either at the eyebrow centre, the nosetip, or a point outside of the body, immediately and beneficially affects the brain, and this has a reciprocal effect on the eye movements, the retina and the whole visual apparatus. Those who have a turbulent mind should practise trataka.

How does trataka affect the mind?

Swami Satyananda: Trataka develops the power of concentration enormously, which is of immense use in everyday life. By stopping the fluctuating tendency of the mind, the mental energy is focused towards one point, leading to peace of mind. Trataka is an excellent method of obtaining meditation experience and unleashing some of the dormant potential of the mind.

The power of memory is hampered in many people by mental disturbances, which seem to cloud over the ability to recall events. Trataka improves the memory by calming the mind.

In India, trataka is often used as a means to gain psychic powers such as telepathy and clairvoyance, but practising for this reason is not recommended, whether one believes in these powers or not, as they are a distraction on the path to higher awareness and self-knowledge.

How does trataka help one harness the power of the mind?

Swami Satyananda: Under the normal waking conditions of life, one is subjected to a continuous stream of sensory data from the outside world. Added to this are the multitudes of thoughts that arise from the subconscious mind, many in response to negative emotions and reactions to inner and external events. Due to this, the enormous power and potential of the mind is not used. Instead the mind operates at a low level compared to its fullest potential. Its energy is dissipated in all directions. Trataka cuts off this continual bombardment of the mind by fixing the attention or field of awareness at one point. In this way one is able to become aware of the potential of the mind, for it spontaneously shows itself under these ideal conditions of concentration. Trataka is a method of consolidating the power of the mind, so that it can be directed towards some useful end, whether material, mental or spiritual.

How does trataka improve concentratration?

Swami Satyananda: Trataka makes the mind steady and helps it to concentrate. When an individual does any intellectual work, listens carefully to something, or thinks, his eyes remain steady, without a flicker, and thus a natural state of trataka is attained. This faculty can be applied consciously by an individual whenever he chooses to do so.

When one wants the mind to be concentrated, trataka should be performed on any object, or inner trataka may be done. For this reason, trataka should be practised for at least five minutes before performing any sadhana. Students should definately practise trataka, as daily practice helps develop the power of concentration, as well as improving memory and eyesight.

How can trataka help students study more effectively?

Swami Niranjanananda: Trataka is the most effective yoga practice for developing concentration. During exam time, trataka on a candle flame should be done for five minutes before beginning studies. Do this for five minutes before going to sleep and before beginning studies. After a couple of days it will be easier to memorize and retain whatever is read. This practice develops mental concentration. It is most important for success in studies.

How can trataka help in the expansion of consciousness?

Swami Satyananda: When trataka is practised, one develops a vision without an object. This requires a greater capacity of mind. After all, sensory objects are not the only reality: one must stop and think again, is there nothing existing beyond all this? Is there no form behind the form? Is there no sound behind the sound? Yes there is, and that experience can be lasting.

It is stated clearly in the Upanishads that sensory experiences are limited by time and space and maya. Only when one can cross over the barrier of sensorial experiences can one come to a deeper reality. This is also the premise of modern psychology. The highest experiences emanate from the unconscious, and the lower spring from maya. Therefore, the practice of trataka is of great relevance in the expansion of consciousness.

How does trataka help purge the unconscious mind?

Swami Satyananda: Karma cannot be dealt with by a rational process such as psychoanalysis or psychiatric treatment, rather it has to be understood as a subtle force underlying each and every action or event that is encountered. The practice of concentration on a symbol is effective in purging these archetypes from the unconscious mind. In yoga this practice of concentration is known as trataka, and it should be done prior to the practice of yoga nidra.

When trataka is practised on a symbol, samskaras are stimulated in the brain. There are hundreds of symbols prescribed in yoga and tantra, out of which some are considered more powerful than others. For example, the effect of concentration on a yantra or mandala depends on the quality inherent in the yantra or mandala. Trataka done on the kali yantra or mandala will bring out repressions more quickly, often in the form of nightmarish experiences. Concentration on other yantras and mandalas brings out a different quantity and quality of repressions. These repressions can be experienced in dreams, or in the state of meditation, and that means the whole samskara is being flushed out. Therefore, side by side with yoga nidra, concentration should be taught according to the quality and resistance of the aspirant.

What are the mental and emotional benefits of trataka?

Swami Niranjanananda: Vision has a direct link with the state of consciousness. Conflicting thoughts lead to mental restlessness and instability. Trataka is the best way to manage this condition. By stabilizing the eyes during trataka the consciousness, *chitta*, can be made steady and free of tension. When the chitta becomes one-pointed, the pineal gland is energized and a higher state is achieved.

Trataka is a simple way to increase memory. It is useful for people suffering from insomnia and nervous tension. Trataka builds self-confidence. It also influences the brainwaves, which change according to one's physical, mental and emotional activities. The frequency of these waves slowly reduces with trataka. The mind becomes thoughtless and free from disorders, and freedom from emotional ailments is attained. The practice increases awareness and calms all dimensions of inner activity, thus releasing energy.

What are the mental and spiritual effects of trataka?

Swami Niranjanananda: Trataka's most important effect is on ajna chakra and the brain. Trataka unlocks the inherent energy of the mind and channels it in the dormant areas of consciousness. Other results of a one-pointed mind are strong willpower, and improved memory and concentration. Trataka is a process of concentrating the mind and curbing its oscillating tendencies. The purpose is to make the mind completely one-pointed and to arouse inner vision.

One-pointed concentration of mind is called *ekagrata*. There are numerous distractions which obstruct ekagrata. In fact, distraction only occurs when the senses are tuned to the external world, which means an energy leakage is occurring.

Association and identification through the eyes are major contributing factors to this leakage.

Furthermore, the eyes constantly move either in large movements, or tremors. Even when the eyes are focused on an external object, the view perceived is always fluctuating due to these spontaneous movements. When the same object is constantly seen, the brain becomes accustomed or habituated and soon stops registering that object. Habituation coincides with an increase in alpha waves, indicating diminished visual attention to the external world. When alpha waves are produced, particular areas of the brain cease functioning.

Vision depends not only on the eyes, but upon the entire optic system. The lens of the eye is only the medium of external visual perception. Via the lens, an image is projected onto the retina. This is a stimulus which excites the retina to fire impulses back to the visual cortex of the brain where an inner image is mapped out. If the eyes are closed and then gently pushed and released, one sees flashes of light, not because light is entering the eyes, but due to stimulation of the optic nerve.

When the image of an external object is stabilized on the retina, after a period of time, perception of the image will completely disappear and a suspension of the mental processes will occur. In fact, if there is absolutely no visual stimulus, for example, if one sits in a pitch dark room or covers the eyes with opaque cups, after some time the mind will turn off just as in sleep. Therefore, during the practice of trataka it is essential to maintain inner awareness so that when the mind is suspended all that remains is the awareness. This is not only in relation to trataka but to any practice of concentration. When the awareness is restricted to one unchanging sensory stimulus, like touch or sound, the mind turns off. Complete absorption in a single perception induces withdrawal of contact with the external world.

Trataka results in a blanking out of visual perception and in the wake of this suspension the central nervous system begins to function in isolation. This experience is known by yogis as sushumna awakening. When the brain is isolated from the sense modalities and the associated mental processes, ideas, memories, etc., triggered by these thought impressions, the spiritual consciousness emerges. The higher mind, liberated from time and space, is experienced. Sushumna is awakened.

What is meant by the attainment of divine vision through practising trataka?

Swami Niranjanananda: In *Gheranda Samhita* it says that through the practice of trataka, *divya drishtih prajayate*, divine vision is achieved. *Divya drishti* means *antar drishti,* inner vision. Symbolically, the inner eye is called the third eye, or the eye of Shiva. It is ajna chakra, where prana shakti and chitta shakti meet and become one. In this sattwic, balanced state they travel up to sahasrara to meet the Supreme Consciousness, Shiva.

From mooladhara to ajna chakra, ida and pingala nadis intersect at each chakra, but they become one on meeting at ajna chakra, which means that from ajna chakra the experience of monism begins: 'I' and 'That' are one. Up to ajna chakra the experience of duality continues: 'I am experiencing this. I am seeing this. I can see the future. I can see the past. I am seeing the present. I can read the thoughts of others. There is the power of attraction in my glance', and so on. This type of experience, and these feelings, remain until the *pancha tattwas,* the five elements, are transcended.

The domain of the five elements is from mooladhara to vishuddhi, and when one rises above these, what can be called knowledge of a sixth sense is attained. In yogic language this sixth sense is antar drishti, inner vision, the establishment of the link or relationship with one's own ishta or guru. With the experience of inner contact and oneness, one becomes the knower of the past, present and future. This is also called divine vision.

Are there examples of advanced souls practising trataka?

Swami Satyananda: The sadhana of trataka helps one understand the mind, making its unseen powers active, in preparation for self-realization. The practice of trataka stands alone, and is meant for aspirants of higher categories; trataka is a powerful sadhana. Queen Gandhari, the wife of King Dhritarashtra of the *Mahabharata*, mastered trataka. Ramana Maharshi also practised trataka. Many sadhus in the mountains practise this sadhana. Trataka sadhana has shown that the eyes are the instruments by which the mind and the soul are reached.

Why is trataka such a powerful sadhana?

Swami Satyananda: Trataka does not merely increase perception; through the medium of perception, the inactive centres of the brain are awakened. There are different categories of people. Man is capable of being a superman if he is able to awaken and activate those glands and nerve centres which in the natural course of evolution are in an inactive state.

Some yogis live in the Himalayas, perform penances and attain siddhis. What practices do they perform? They perform sadhanas through which they develop the inner centres of the body. Thus, their senses are fully developed. These things are not impossible, they are natural, rational, intelligible and form part of evolution. Every person who can devote the time can practise them under the guidance of a guru.

In brief, what are the benefits of trataka?

Swami Niranjanananda: Sage Gheranda succinctly lists the benefits of trataka in *Gheranda Samhita* (1:54). First, *netrarogaa vinashyanti*, trataka removes defects of the eyes. This is its physical benefit. Second, *divyadrishtih prajaayate*, divine vision is created. This is its divine benefit. Third, *shaambhavee jaayate dhruvam*, the siddhi of shambhavi is achieved. This is its spiritual benefit.

TRATAKA AND MEDITATION

How can trataka lead to meditation?

Swami Sivananda: When one gazes at a picture, it is trataka. When one closes the eyes and mentally visualizes the picture, it is *saguna dhyana*, meditation with form. Meditation is an unbroken, uninterrupted or incessant flow of the idea of the object that is concentrated upon. In the beginning, concrete meditation on an object is necessary for an untrained mind.

When one associates with the attributes of God such as omnipresence, omnipotence, omniscience, purity and perfection, the name and form of the object of trataka will automatically disappear and *nirguna dhyana*, abstract meditation will be entered into. If one meditates on an abstract idea, it is *nirguna* meditation.

What is the link between meditation and trataka?

Swami Satyananda: Trataka is a most powerful practice for developing concentration. It is also an excellent method of developing inner visualization; in other words the ability to see and maintain a clear image of any object in front of the closed eyes. Both of these abilities are important for meditation.

In the practice of trataka the mind is directed towards an external object such as a dot, the flame of a candle, a picture of a cross, *Om*, or anything in fact. However, it is best to choose an object that has deep meaning for the practitioner. This helps to hold the mind more firmly on the object of concentration. The object should also be something that the eyes can easily focus on and which does not disturb the mind. Whatever the object, it has the same function: to 'trap' all the attention of the mind and eyes and focus it on one point. This sounds simple, but in fact it creates some difficulty for most people as their minds are accustomed to jumping from one thought to the next.

After concentration on the object, the eyes are closed and the practitioner tries to visualize an inner image of the external object. Inner concentration is preferable to external concentration for meditation practices, as it further reduces the tendency of the mind to wander. However, inner trataka is more difficult than external trataka, as a distinct image must be visualized. Ideally it is a non-changing image for the duration of the concentration, for if it fades or disappears the depth of concentration is lost. Practice is required. Everyone, with dedication and regularity in practice can eventually master this technique.

Why is concentration so important in yoga?

Swami Satyananda: It is through powerful concentration that one makes progress in yoga, and concentration is the essence of trataka. What is concentration? It is one-pointedness of mind, the ability to hold, to focus one's attention on one point, without wavering. Perfect concentration leads to meditation. In meditation practices, such as trataka, concentration leads to complete mental attention on one object, form or thought to the exclusion of all others. There is no distraction from the environment or other peripheral experiences.

In recent years science has produced something that was once a topic of science fiction novels – the laser. It is an apparatus that lines up all the rays of light from a source so that they are in unison with each other, so that they vibrate together in perfect harmony. The original source of light need not be great, not even as great as the average light bulb filament, yet if one stood five feet away from a laser source, the beam would almost instantaneously burn a hole straight through one's body. This is the power of concentrated light.

Concentrated thought, though unlikely to bore a hole in the body, also has vast power. A concentrated mind acts as an irresistible instrument of action; it leads to efficiency in all one's activities in the outside world; it is a dynamo which generates vitality and enthusiasm in every direction. A concentrated mind also has the ability to be a sensitive receiving instrument; it becomes receptive to higher vibrations, to heightened perception. It becomes a receiver of the influx of higher awareness, bliss and knowledge. All this is normally beyond the range of the average mind for it is too disturbed and distracted by a continual inner chatter of thoughts. Concentration is the key that will unlock the door to higher states of awareness.

Is trataka more than an effort of concentration?

Swami Niranjanananda: In trataka, apart from concentrating the mind, one has to witness what is happening in the mind from moment to moment. Concentration of mind is an external act which one tries to perform. The sadhaka forces himself to sit straight and still, to gaze until the eyes begin to water, then closing the eyes he tries to hold the image inside. That is an effort of concentration, but apart from that effort there is the awareness that one is trying to align oneself. It is this awareness which enables one to hold onto that point of concentration and witness what is happening within the mind. Ultimately that is the result which is aimed for in trataka.

Is trataka a technique of dharana?

Swami Niranjanananda: Trataka is a technique of dharana which focuses the mind on one point or one object of concentration. After the relaxation of the uncontrolled and unchannelled physical, mental and pranic activities, one goes into a state of concentration with the practice of trataka.

Trataka means 'to see', 'to look at'. Visual perception is the most powerful *indriya* or sensory organ in this manifest world. It is possible to see for miles and miles, to perceive what is happening many miles away, without actually being there. In trataka it is the vision that is focused. To achieve concentration, the visual distractions which affect concentration and awareness must be minimized: this is done through the practice of trataka, steady gazing.

How does trataka lead to dhyana?

Swami Niranjanananda: When dharana becomes steady during trataka on a candle flame, it can lead to dhyana. In dhyana, the candle flame appears with dimensions. With dharana on an object with dimensions, dhyana begins, as there is no difference between what is seen internally in dhyana and what is seen in external life. If an object is seen in dhyana it is as real as it would be in actual life; there is three-dimensional awareness. In the practice of trataka on an object with dimensions, that vivid awareness has to be developed if it is to take one into dhyana.

PREPARATION FOR HIGHER SADHANA

What type of visions occur during trataka?

Swami Sivananda: The object of gazing may appear as something else during the practice. There may be many visions. Different people have different experiences. Some things cannot be believed when others tell of their experiences.

Does trataka help develop the willpower needed in higher sadhana?

Swami Sivananda: Trataka lies at the base of willpower. It is a preliminary sadhana for a yogic student. A jnani concentrates his attention on an abstract thought, such as, *Aham Brahmasmi*; 'I am all purity. I am all power.' It is uphill work, it is a tremendous task for the average person to concentrate on an abstract thought; to begin with, one must concentrate on a concrete object.

How does trataka become a higher sadhana?

Swami Niranjanananda: In the practice of trataka, when there is awareness of the viewer, the view and the process of viewing, fears begin to be destroyed gradually, one by one. It has been noticed that when people start practising trataka after having performed yogic practices for a long period, then as one fear arises and ends, a second one arises and ends, then a third one arises and ends. This process continues.

In hatha yoga it is believed that by merely practising trataka a person can become a master of all siddhis and can attain the state of self-realization, as the mind merges into the object. Trataka can therefore be considered as a practice of *laya yoga*, where the practitioner's consciousness dissolves into whatever is concentrated upon.

It is essential to choose an external form for *bahir* or external trataka. As stated earlier, trataka can be practised on anything, whether it is a flame, one's own shadow or some other symbol. After practising trataka on the external object or symbol, one may enter into subtle or internal antar trataka. Once this is perfected, practices such as shambhavi mudra take on a different dimension.

How can trataka be used for developing sensitivity to ajna chakra?

Swami Satyananda: Trataka is a powerful technique. With regard to developing sensitivity to the location of ajna chakra and bhrumadhya, a candle is certainly the best object. When gazing at the candle, or whatever object is chosen, the feeling should be as though one is gazing with the eyebrow centre instead of the two eyes.

A particularly powerful method for simultaneously developing sensitivity to both ajna and bhrumadhya involves the integration of trataka with the flow of breath. One tries to feel that the breath is piercing both ajna and bhrumadhya while it flows to and fro along the maha nadi. That is, with the inhalation there is a feeling that the breath is being drawn in through the eyebrow centre to eventually pierce ajna; and with the exhalation, there is a feeling that the breath is being pushed forwards from ajna to eventually pierce the eyebrow centre. This type of awareness continues while maintaining a concentrated gaze on the candle flame.

What is the role of trataka in the awakening of ajna chakra?

Swami Niranjanananda: With the awakening of ajna chakra, the dormant layers of the mind are stimulated. With the awakening of these dormant areas, the distinction in the perceptions of what is conscious, what is subconscious and what is unconscious disappears. This change takes place at the level of ajna chakra. *Bodh*, enlightenment, mental awakening, takes place at the level of ajna chakra. That state of awakening has to be channelled, and that is done through the practice of trataka. The sixth practice of hatha yoga is trataka, which is a way of achieving optimum concentration of awareness and mind.

What does the experience of becoming one with the flame during trataka mean?

Swami Niranjanananda: That is the state of *dhyana*, total identification with the object of concentration. It is an excellent state of mind to achieve, as in normal life there is always a disassociation between awareness and experience. Any experience can be observed, but if through some method the practitioner can become one with the experience or the event that is taking place within, that becomes the state of dhyana. This experience should be intensified with further sadhana.

Can kundalini be awakened through regular practise of trataka?

Swami Satyananda: The sleeping kundalini resides in mooladhara and its path of ascent is through sushumna nadi. Unless one has been a regular practitioner of yoga for some time, ida and pingala are not in communication with sushumna. But when trataka and kapalbhati are practised, these nadis are connected; when this link is established, the higher energy flows through them.

What effect does trataka have on the pranas and the mind?

Swami Niranjanananda: The different forms of trataka, such as concentration on the moon, a star, a candle flame or a crystal, help to focus and channel the pranic energies. When these energies are channelled, the entire mental framework is influenced. The mind becomes stable and balanced and begins to function more efficiently.

Why should the mind be emptied of thoughts during trataka?

Swami Niranjanananda: In the initial practice of trataka, when one begins to concentrate intently on the object, the dissipated mind becomes focused in concentration. As long as external trataka is practised the mind remains steady and concentration remains sharp, even though after trataka the normal dissipated nature of the mind returns. During the practice, however, the pratyahara of the senses induces the pratyahara of the mental faculties, leading to dharana of the mental faculties, which is known as antaranga trataka. Holding the mental faculties at one point of concentration and not allowing them to waver is the subtle aspect of trataka.

When trataka is described in *Hatha Yoga Pradipika* (2:31), Yogi Swatmarama speaks of *sukshma lakshya* or 'the subtle direction'. According to yoga this means awareness of the mental faculties and holding the concentration of the mental faculties rather than the normal concentration on the sensory perceptions. It is here that keeping the mind entirely devoid of thought helps one pinpoint and bring together the states of manas, buddhi and chitta.

In the practice of antaranga trataka, manas, buddhi and chitta, the three mental faculties, are centred in the object of concentration. Unless the concentration becomes so intense that there is no separation of 'me' as the practitioner and the object and process of practice, one cannot experience the higher states, one cannot experience samadhi, and one cannot go beyond the state of *ahamkara* – ego. In *Sri Vijnana Bhairava Tantra* (v. 80) this is described:

> *Sthoolaroopasya bhavasya stabdhaam drishtam nipaatya cha*
> *Achirena niraadhaaram manah kritvaa shivam vrajet.*

One should steady the gaze (without blinking) on the gross form of any object. When the mind is transfixed and made supportless (without any other thought or feeling), it at once acquires the state of shiva (transcendence).

What is the purpose of practising trataka on a yantra?

Swami Niranjanananda: Focusing on an external image of a yantra can take the practitioner into a deeper level of the mind, giving access to one's own internal yantra.

Why is trataka associated with shambhavi mudra?

Swami Niranjanananda: In *Gheranda Samhita* (1:54) it is said that it is essential to have mastery over trataka in order to perfect shambhavi mudra:

Evamabhyaasayogena shaambhavee jaayate dhruvam;
Netrarogaa vinashyanti divyadrishtih prajaayate.

With constant practice of trataka, shambhavi mudra is achieved, defects of the eyes are removed and divine vision is attained.

Shambhavi mudra is an apparently simple practice in which one looks at the eyebrow centre. It should be understood that when shambhavi is perfected, *shambhavi siddhi*, control over the subtle elements, is achieved. This siddhi is illustrated by a story from the *Puranas*, the ancient scriptures.

Sati, the consort of Shiva, attended a *yajna*, a ceremonial fire sacrifice, in the kingdom of her father, Daksha. She noticed that Lord Shiva had not been invited and in response to this insult, she self-immolated, reducing her body to ashes. She is described as sitting in an asana and focusing her vision at the eyebrow centre. Keeping her

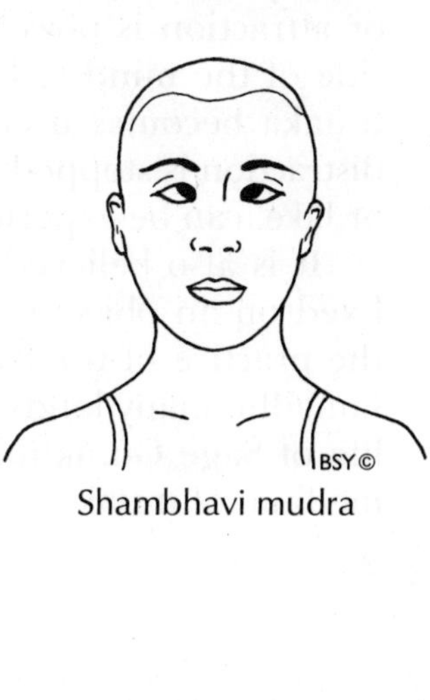

Shambhavi mudra

ishta in the heart centre, she reduced her body to ashes by yogic fire.

Shaambhavee jaayate dhruvam, shambhavi siddhi is attained. Thus it has been described in both the ancient scriptures and modern yogic texts that with shambhavi siddhi, yogis attain control over the subtle elements. When this is achieved, a person becomes omniscient and omnipotent.

How does practising trataka help one to maintain the state of samadhi?

Swami Niranjanananda: Through the practice of trataka one can develop the ability to focus the mind at any time, a necessary skill in the higher practices of yoga. There is a deep meaning behind the practice of trataka. Sage Patanjali's *Yoga Sutras* declare that even in the highest state of meditation or samadhi, certain impressions, ideas or experiences remain in the consciousness, and thus they disturb the concentration of mind. These deep impressions or ideas which do not disappear, even in samadhi, are known as *pratyaya*. Trataka is considered to be the best practice for clearing and purifying the *antahkarana*, the inner tool of consciousness.

If the mind has not been taught to concentrate and concentration has only been practised superficially, when these pratyaya manifest in deep meditative states their pull or attraction is powerful, as there is nothing on the other side of the mind to balance it. The ability gained through trataka becomes useful at that moment. When the visual distraction is stopped, a quiet mind, which is like a still pond or lake, can be experienced.

It is also believed that when the antahkarana becomes fixed on an object or a symbol and merges with it during the practice of trataka, laya samadhi is attained. With laya samadhi, many kinds of siddhis arise. This was noted in the life of Sage Gorakhnath who attained siddhis through the medium of trataka.

What happens when trataka becomes a complete experience?

Swami Satyananda: Trataka is a powerful, yet deceptively simple practice. When one is able to concentrate on an object, that object becomes the focus and the form of one's consciousness. In other words, if the object is a candle, it does not merely represent one's consciousness, it is one's consciousness. This is hard to understand, but it is worth pointing out. All one has to do is practise trataka and merge one's being into the object, form or thought, disappearing into it like an arrowhead into a target.

To accomplish this, any method of trataka can be practised, according to one's liking. Achieve the knowledge of yoga and the spiritual science with your own experience. There is nothing higher than self-experience and there is no joy greater than the joy of practising sadhana.

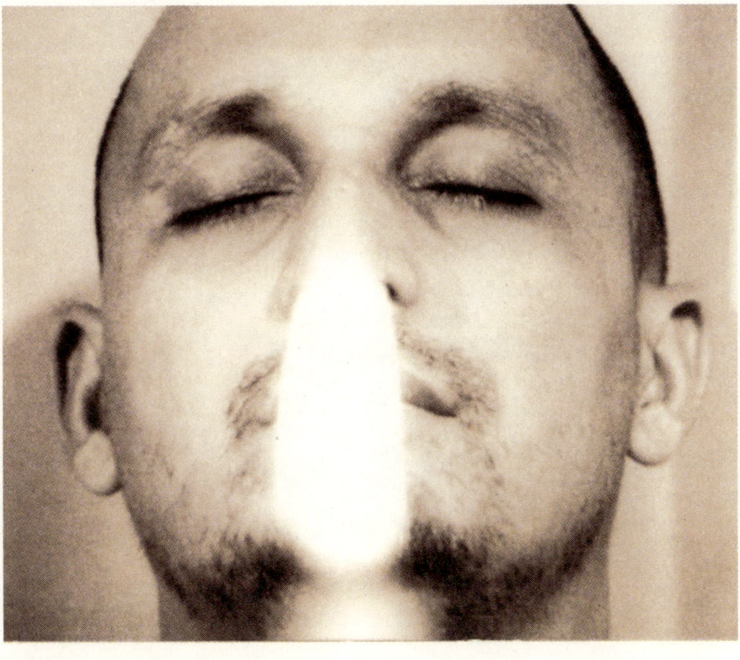

Appendices

Appendix A

Index of Questions

1. Understanding the Shatkarmas

DEFINITION AND CLASSIFICATION

3. Neti: Nasal Cleansing

GUIDELINES FOR PRACTICE

BENEFITS

ATTAINMENTS

8. Basti: Yogic Enema

Appendix B

Index of Scriptural Quotes

BHAGAVAD GITA

11. Trataka: Steady gazing

(6:26) From whatever cause the restless, unsteady mind wanders away, from that let him restrain it and bring it under the control of the Self alone. 204

GHERANDA SAMHITA

1. Understanding the Shatkarmas

(1:10) Through shatkarmas purification of body and through asanas firmness, through mudras steadiness and through pratyahara patience is achieved. 18

3. Neti: Nasal Cleansing

(1:51) The practice of neti enables one to attain perfection in khechari, elimination of kapha and attainment of divine vision. 38, 56

(1:50) Take a thread half as long as the arm, insert it in the nose and take it out through the mouth. This is called neti karma. 56

4. Introduction to Dhauti

(1:13) Antar dhauti, danta dhauti, hrid dhauti and moola shodhana are the four types of dhauti which keep the body clean and healthy. 58

5. Antar Dhauti: Internal Cleansing

(1:15) Shaping the lips like a crow's beak, slowly, slowly suck in as much air as possible, circulate it inside the abdomen and then gradually expel it completely. 65

(1:16) Vatsara is a very secret technique for purifying the body. It destroys all diseases and activates the gastric fire, which helps to digest food. 68

(1:17) Drink water slowly through the mouth up to the throat. The abdomen is then moved and the water evacuated through the anus. 71

(1:18) The technique of varisara dhauti is most secret. It purifies the body. A yogi who perfects this technique attains a divine body. 71

(1:19) Retaining prana vayu, pull the navel against the spinal column one hundred times. This enables agnisara dhauti to be performed. Diseases of the abdomen are removed and the digestive fire is stimulated. 88

(1:20) This cleansing practice is most secret and is unknown even to the divine beings. By merely doing this practice the body becomes healthy and beautiful, there is no doubt about that. 89

(1:22) Standing in water up to the navel, push out the rectum (shakti nadi) and wash it, removing the waste products. When the nadi is clean, draw it in again. 94

(1:23) This cleansing practice of dhauti is very secret. It is not even accessible to the gods. Just by practising this dhauti, one attains a body like that of a divine being. 94

(1:24) It is not possible to practise bahishkrita mahadhauti until the ability to retain air in the abdomen for up to one and a half hours has been developed. 94

(1:21) Purse the lips like the beak of a crow, take in air through the mouth, filling the abdomen. Retain the air for one and a half hours in the abdomen, then circulate it and expel it through the rectum. It is top secret and is called bahishkrita dhauti. 95

(1:42) Cruel (disorders of apana vayu) cannot be removed without performing moola shodhana (anal cleansing). 105

(1:43) Cleaning of the anus is essential with a turmeric root or the middle finger combined with repeated washing with water. 105

(1:44)This practice removes hard faeces and constipation, the body becomes graceful and healthy and the digestive fire is stimulated. 105

6. Danta Dhauti: Head Cleansing

(1:25) There are five kinds of danta dhauti: dantamoola (cleaning the teeth), jihvamoola (cleaning the tongue), karnarandhra (cleaning the two ears) and kapalarandhra (cleaning the upper region of the head). Thus there are five in all. 107

(1:26) Rub or massage the roots of the teeth with the juice of the khadira plant (Acacia catechu) or with clean earth until the impurities are removed. 109

(1:27) Yogis must adopt this method every morning to protect their teeth. Those who know yoga consider dantamoola dhauti to be a significant part of the purification process. 109

(1:28) Now I will tell you the method for cleaning the tongue. Lengthening of the tongue destroys old age, death and disease. 112

(1:29) The root of the tongue should be cleaned by inserting the index finger, middle finger and ring finger in the throat. Kapha disorders (phlegm) are removed by slowly and gently rubbing the tongue. 112

(1:30) Once this cleaning and rubbing is over, apply a little butter on the tongue. Again perform the action like that of milking a cow. Thereafter, stretch the tongue out with the help of small tongs. 113

(1:31)The length of the tongue increases by doing this practice daily at the time of sunrise and sunset. 113

(1:32) Clean the orifices of both ears with the index and ring fingers. By practising this daily, nada or inner sound may be heard. 115

(1:33) Massage the forehead with the right hand thumb. With this type of practice one is relieved of kapha dosha. 119

(1:34)The nadis are purified and divine vision is attained. Practise daily at the end of sleep, after food and before sleep. 119

7. Hrid Dhauti: Cleansing the Heart Region

(1:35) There are three types of hrid dhauti: using a stick, regurgitating water, and using cloth. 121

(1:36) The stem of a soft portion of the banana tree, a thin turmeric stem or a sugarcane stem should be repeatedly inserted (through the mouth) and then slowly withdrawn from the middle chest. 122

10. Kapalbhati: Frontal Brain Cleansing

(1:55) Vatakrama, vyutkrama and sheetkrama are the three types of bhalbhati. Practising them eliminates phlegm and mucus from the body. 173

(1:56) The breath is to be inhaled through ida nadi (the left nostril) and exhaled through pingala nadi (the right nostril). Then the breath is inhaled through surya nadi (the right nostril) and exhaled through chandra nadi (the left nostril). 175

(1:57) Inhalation and exhalation should be fast; do not hold it. This technique removes kapha dosha. 175

(1:58) Suck water through both nostrils and expel it through the mouth. Practise this repeatedly. This vyutkrama kapalbhati removes kapha disorders. 177

(1:59) Suck in water through the mouth with a hissing sound and expel it through the nose. Through this practice the body of the practitioner becomes as beautiful as that of Kamadeva, the god of love. 179

(1:60) Signs of old age do not manifest. Cleanliness and purity manifest in the body and kapha dosha is removed. 179

11. Trataka: Steady gazing

(1:53) Gazing at a subtle object without blinking the eyes, until tears begin to fall, is known as trataka. 188

(1:54) With constant practice of trataka, shambhavi mudra is achieved, defects of the eyes are removed and divine vision is attained. 241

HATHA YOGA PRADIPIKA

1. Understanding the Shatkarmas

(2:23) These shatkarmas which effect purification of the body are secret. They have manifold, wondrous results and are held in high esteem by eminent yogis. 16

(2:36) By the six karmas, (shatkarmas), one is freed from excesses of the doshas. Pranayama can then be practised and success achieved without strain. 21

2. Shatkarma Sadhana

(2:21) When fat or mucus is excessive, shatkarma: the six cleansing techniques, should be practised before (pranayama). Others, in whom the doshas, i.e. phlegm, wind and bile, are balanced should not do them. 31

(2:37) According to some teachers, pranayama alone removes impurities and therefore they hold pranayama in esteem and not the other techniques. 35

3. Neti: Nasal Cleansing

(2:29) Insert a soft thread through the nose to the length of one handspan so that it comes out of the mouth. This is called neti by the siddhas. 40

4. Introduction to Dhauti

(2:25) There is no doubt that coughs, asthma, diseases of the spleen, leprosy and twenty kinds of diseases caused by excess mucus are destroyed through the effects of dhauti karma. 60

7. Hrid Dhauti: Cleansing the Heart Region

(2:38) Vomiting the things in the stomach by moving the apana into the throat is called gaja karani by those who have attained knowledge of hatha yoga. Becoming accustomed to this technique, brings about control of the nadis and chakras. 134

(2:24) A strip of wet cloth, four angulas wide (seven to eight centimetres) and fifteen handspans (one and a half metres) in length is slowly swallowed and then taken out, as instructed by the guru. This is known as dhauti. 135

8. Basti: Yogic Enema

(2:26) Sitting in utkatasana, navel deep in water, insert a tube into the anus and contract the anus. This cleansing with water is called basti karma. 151

(2:27) Enlargement of the glands and spleen, and all diseases arising from excess wind, bile and mucus are eliminated from the body through the practice of basti. 154

(2:28) By practising jala basti the appetite increases, the body glows, excess doshas are destroyed and the dhatu, senses and mind are purified. 155

9. Nauli: Abdominal Massage

(2:34) Nauli is foremost of the hatha yoga practices. It kindles the digestive fire, removing indigestion, sluggish digestion, and all disorders of the doshas, and brings about happiness. 169

10. Kapalbhati: Frontal Brain Cleansing

(2:35) Perform exhalation and inhalation rapidly like the bellows (of a blacksmith). This is called kapalbhati; it destroys all mucous disorders. 172

11. Trataka: Steady gazing

(2:31) Looking intently with an unwavering gaze at a small point until tears are shed is known as trataka by the acharyas (teachers). 187

HATHARATNAVALI

1. Understanding the Shatkarmas

(1:25) Now I will speak on the eight karmas according to the guru tradition: chakri, nauli, dhauti, neti, basti, gajakarani, trataka and mastakabhati (kapalabhati), these are said to be eight purificatory processes. 12

(1:59) These eight purificatory processes purify the six chakras thoroughly and all types of diseases are destroyed. It is the way to attain moksha and also the base for practising pranayama. 28

(1:61) The base is purified through chakri karma and the male organ is purified through vajroli karma. 28

(1:62) Manipura, situated in the navel region, is purified through the karma named nauli. 29

(1:63) The chakra situated in the region of the heart and throat is purified through the karma named dhauti. 29

(1:64) Purification of ajna chakra is done through neti and trataka karmas. 29

(1:29) Piles, diseases of the spleen and distended stomach are cured; evacuation of the bowels, and stimulation of the digestive fire take place through chakrikarma. 104

8. Basti: Yogic Enema

(1:41) Basti is said to be of two types: water and air. After doing chakrikarma according to the best of one's effort, one should practise basti. 143

(1:42) After collecting air in the stomach, release it through the lower passage (anus). Vayu basti is explained; Now I will speak about jala basti. 144

(1:43) Now jala basti: Standing in water up to the navel region, put the finger in the passage of the anus. Through the chakri process, the stomach should be filled with water through the anus. 144

(1:44) Then, after doing vichitra karani, one should draw out the water without fear. Draw the water according to your strength, wait for some moments then expel it. 144

(1:45) After practising basti one should not take a meal for three ghatis (seventy two minutes). He should sit peacefully on the ground and take controlled, pleasurable and moderate food. 153

9. Nauli: Abdominal Massage

(1:32) With shoulders bent forward one should rotate the abdomen (muscles) right and left with the speed of a fast rotating whirlpool. This nauli is praised by the accomplished yogis. 159

(1:34) Fast rotation from ida and then again from pingala; rotation of these two is called antara nauli according to me. 164

(1:33) Nauli the crown of hatha practices, makes the gastric fire blaze up, improves digestion etc., invariably brings a feeling of wellbeing and completely destroys all disorders and diseases. 168

10. Kapalbhati: Frontal Brain Cleansing

(1:54) Now kapalbhati: Rapid performance of inhalation and exhalation like the bellows of the blacksmith is kapalbhati, well known as the destroyer of all diseases. 175

(1:55) Fast rotation of breathing from left to right and right to left, and exhalation and inhalation is called kapalbhati. 175

11. Trataka: Steady gazing

(1:52) Now trataka: Well composed and keeping the sight steady, one should stare at a small object until tears come out. This is called trataka by the teachers. 222

(1:53) Trataka, which clears eye diseases and prevents sloth should be valued and kept secret with the same effort as one keeps a casket of precious stones. 223

SRI VIJNANA BHAIRAVA TANTRA

11. Trataka: Steady gazing

(v. 80) One should steady the gaze (without blinking) on the gross form of any object. When the mind is transfixed and made supportless (without any other thought or feeling), it at once acquires the state of shiva (transcendence). 241

Glossary

Agni – fire; the god of fire.

Aham Brahmasmi – 'I am Brahman', one of the four great vedic statements known as maha vakya.

Ahamkara – faculty of ego, awareness of the existence of 'I'; one of the four parts of the antahkarana or inner instrument.

Ajna chakra – psychic/pranic centre situated at the medulla oblongata at the top of the spinal column in the mid-brain; seat of intuition, higher knowledge; third eye.

Amavasya – no moon.

Amrita – the nectar of immortality which descends from bindu.

Anahata chakra – psychic/pranic centre situated in the spine behind the sternum; associated physically with the cardiac plexus, heart and lungs, mentally with emotion, especially love, and spiritually with atma, the spirit.

Anandamaya kosha – sheath or body of bliss; the innermost wrapper or sheath of the embodied spirit.

Anga – limb.

Annamaya kosha – sheath or body of matter; the sphere of existence created by food, maintained by food and which ultimately becomes food, i.e. the body.

Antah, antar – inner.

Antahkarana – literally, 'inner tool', inner organ of consciousness, consisting of: ahamkara, manas, buddhi and chitta.

Antaranga – inner part; internal portion.
Antaryamin – inner ruler; the Supreme Being present in every object of creation and guiding all creatures.
Apana vayu – one of the pancha pranas or vayus, it is located between the navel and the perineum. It flows downward and controls elimination and reproduction.
Ardha chakrasana – half-wheel pose; a backward bending asana.
Asana – a specific yoga posture; used in hatha yoga to channel prana, open the chakras and remove energy blocks; in raja yoga, a physical posture in which one is at ease and in harmony with oneself.
Ashtanga yoga – the eight limbs of yoga described by Sage Patanjali in the *Yoga Sutras*: yama, niyama, asana, pranayama, pratyahara, dharana, dhyana and samadhi.
Ashwini mudra – horse gesture; a yogic practice to redirect energy upwards; mudra involving contraction of the anal sphincter.
Aum – the universal cosmic mantra representing the four states of consciousness; the sound indicating the Supreme Reality or Brahman; conveys concepts of omniscience, omnipresence and omnipotence.
Avarana – ignorance; veiling or covering which hides or excludes part of the reality; a function of maya. See Maya.
Ayurveda – science of health or medicine; the vedic system of medical diagnosis and treatment.
Bahiranga – external part.
Bandha – psycho-muscular energy locks which close the pranic exits (like throat, anus etc); psychic locks that concentrate the flow of energy in the body at one point or plexus.
Basti – one of the shatkarmas; yogic enema.
Bhagavad Gita – literally, 'divine song'; Sri Krishna's discourse to his disciple Arjuna delivered on the battlefield of Kurukshetra at the commencement of the great Mahabharata war; one of the source books of Hindu philosophy, containing the essence of the Upanishads and yoga.

Bhakta – devotee.

Bhakti yoga – branch of yoga in which emotional energy is channelled towards a relationship with the divine; a systematic path with nine stages which expand, strengthen, and purify the emotions.

Bhalarandhra – the forehead; the depression above the nose just above the eyebrow centre.

Bhastrika pranayama – bellows breathing; pranayama in which the breath is forcibly drawn in and out through the nose in equal proportions, like the pumping action of the bellows.

Bhrumadhya – trigger point for ajna chakra located at the eyebrow centre.

Bindu – seed, source, drop; point of potential energy and consciousness, used in kriya yoga; the basis from which emanated the first principle according to the tantra shastra; nucleus; psychic centre located in the brain; in tantra and hatha yoga it also represents a drop of semen.

Bindu visarga – centre or source of individual creation from where psychic vibrations first emanate. See Bindu.

Bodh – enlightenment.

Brahmacharya – being absorbed in higher consciousness; sensual restraint; celibacy; conduct suitable for proceeding to the highest state of existence; one of the yamas described by Sage Patanjali in the *Yoga Sutras* as resulting in indomitable courage.

Brahman – etymologically 'ever expanding, limitless consciousness'; name of Supreme Consciousness or cosmic intelligence according to Vedanta philosophy; God as creator; monistic concept of Absolute Reality.

Brahmarandhra – crown of the head; the fontanelle; opening in the crown of the head through which the soul is said to escape on leaving the body.

Buddhi – discerning, discriminating aspect of the mind; aspect of the mind closest to pure consciousness; one of the four parts of the antahkarana, or inner instrument.

Chakra – circle, wheel or vortex; pranic/psychic centre; confluence point of energy flows (nadis) in the body; the seven major chakras for descent of divine energy or for human evolution are sahasrara, ajna, vishuddhi, anahata, manipura, swadhisthana and mooladhara.

Chakra shodhana – purification of the chakras.

Chakra shuddhi – purification of the chakras.

Chandra shakti – mental force, ida nadi.

Chhaya – shade; reflection.

Chidakasha – the space of consciousness; the inner space visualized in meditation behind the closed eyes or in the region of ajna chakra.

Chinta – thinking, thought; worry, care, anxiety.

Chitta – individual consciousness, including the subconscious and unconscious layers of the mind; thinking, concentration, attention, enquiry; storehouse of memory or samskaras; one of the four parts of the antahkarana, or inner instrument.

Chitta shakti – the power of pure consciousness; mental force governing the subtle dimensions.

Danta – teeth.

Darshan – a glimpse; vision; direct perception; philosophy.

Dussehra – the day on which Sri Rama vanquished Ravana in the Ramayana. It is celebrated the day after Navaratri on the tenth day of the lunar calendar; also called Vijaya Dashami.

Devadeham – a divine, lustrous, brilliant and light body like that of a god.

Devata – form of divine dignity or power; divine being representing the higher states of evolution.

Devi – female deity, goddess.

Dhairya, dhairyam – the fourth limb of Sage Gheranda's saptanga yoga; constancy; steadiness; calmness; patience.

Dharana – practice of concentration or complete attention; sixth stage of ashtanga yoga described in Sage Patanjali's *Yoga Sutras* as holding or binding the mind to one point.

Dhatu – seven constituents of the body: blood, bone, marrow, fat, semen, skin and flesh.

Dhauti – one of the shatkarmas; cleansing techniques for the digestive system, chest and head.

Dhyana – spontaneous state of meditation; one-pointedness of mind through concentration on either a form, thought or sound; absorption in the object of meditation; seventh stage of Sage Patanjali's ashtanga yoga.

Divya drishti – inner vision, divine vision.

Dosha – three humours of the body described in ayurveda: mucus (kapha), bile (pitta) and wind (vata). Their imbalance prevents the flow of energy in sushumna nadi.

Dridhata – the second limb of Sage Gheranda's saptanga yoga; fixed, firm, strong, certain, unshaken.

Ekadashi – 11th day of the lunar fortnight, a time when mantra chanting and dietary restraint are held to be beneficial.

Ekagrata – one-pointedness of mind, fourth of the five states of mind where pure sattwa guna predominates enabling concentrated or meditative states of mind.

Ganesha – the elephant-headed Hindu deity who is the remover of obstacles.

Ghati – time measure equal to 24 minutes.

Gheranda Samhita – traditional text on hatha yoga by Sage Gheranda. It explains seven limbs (saptanga) of yoga: shatkarma, asana, mudra, pratyahara, pranayama, dhyana and samadhi.

Gheranda, Sage – author of Gheranda Samhita, a classical yoga text which describes seven limbs of yoga.

Gorakhnath, Yogi – founder of the Nath sect; author of *Gorakhsha Samhita*.

Guna – quality; the three gunas, qualities or aspects of prakriti are sattwa, rajas and tamas.

Guru – one who dispels the darkness caused by ignorance (avidya); teacher of the science of ultimate reality who by the light of his own atma can dispel darkness, ignorance and illusion from the mind and enlighten the consciousness of a devotee/disciple; preceptor.

Ha – seed mantra of surya shakti.

Hamsasana – swan pose; an advanced yogasana which exerts pressure on the abdominal region.

Hatha yoga – a system of yoga specifically using practices for bodily purification; yoga of attaining physical and mental purity and balancing the prana (energy) in ida and pingala nadis so that sushumna nadi opens, enabling experiences of samadhi. See Ha. See Tha.

Hatha Yoga Pradipika – a major classical text on hatha yoga compiled by Yogi Swatmarama, usually translated as 'Light on Hatha Yoga'.

Hatharatnavali – a late medieval treatise on hatha yoga and tantra by Srinivasa Bhatta Mahayogindra.

Ida nadi – a major pranic channel running from the left side of mooladhara chakra to the left side of ajna chakra, governing the left side of the body and the right side of the brain. The ida energy flow criss-crosses the spine through the major chakras between mooladhara and ajna, conducting the passive aspect of prana manifesting as the mental force, lunar force or chitta shakti; also called chandra nadi, as the lunar energy flows through it.

Indriya – sense organ; power of the senses; power.

Ishta devata – personal deity, one's favourite symbol of the Supreme.

Janmashtami – eighth day of the dark fortnight in the lunar month of Bhadrapada, birthday of Sri Krishna.

Japa – a meditation practice involving repetition of a mantra.

Jatharagni – digestive fire.

Jnani – one who expresses wisdom in daily life.

Jnanendriya – organ of sense perceptions and knowledge; five in number, viz. ears, eyes, nose, tongue and skin.

Jyoti – a small flame; light, brightness; fire.

Jyotirlingam – natural oval-shaped stone worshipped as Lord Shiva; symbol of pure consciousness.

Kagasana – crow pose; a squatting position.

Kaki mudra – the crow's beak; a mudra in which air is inhaled through pursed lips.

Kali – primal manifestation of Shakti; wife of Shiva; deity, divine mother; destroyer of time, space and object, i.e. ignorance.

Kama – emotional, sensual love; lust.

Kamadeva – the god of love.

Kapalarandhra – the upper, slightly hollow region of the head, which can be clearly seen on a newborn baby. See Brahmarandhra.

Kapalbhati – frontal brain cleansing breath; one of the six major cleansing techniques, shatkarmas of hatha yoga; process of purifying the frontal region of the brain by breathing rapidly through the nostrils with emphasis on exhalation.

Kapha – mucus, phlegm, one of the three humours (doshas) described in ayurveda. See Dosha.

Karana sharira – causal body; also called anandamaya kosha.

Karma – action and result; law of cause and effect.

Karma yoga – yogic path of action; union with the Supreme Consciousness through action; action without attachment to the fruits of action.

Karmendriya – motor organ; there are five physical organs of action, viz. vocal cords, hands, feet, genital organ and anus.

Kati chakrasana – waist rotating pose; a dynamic spinal twist; used in shankhaprakshalana.

Kaya – the physical body.

Khechari mudra – literally, 'the attitude of moving in space'; tongue lock; a hatha yoga practice in which the elongated tongue passes back into the pharynx to stimulate the flow of life-giving nectar (amrita), whereas in the milder raja yoga form the tongue is inserted in, or folded backwards towards, the upper cavity of the palate.

Kirtan – singing of God's name; practice in which a group of people sing a collection of mantras.

Kosha – sheath or body; a dimension of experience and existence; the five koshas are: annamaya kosha, pranamaya kosha, manomaya kosha, vijnamaya kosha, and anandamaya kosha.

Krishna, Sri – literally, 'black' or 'dark'; eighth incarnation of Vishnu; avatara who descended in the Dwapara Yuga. Sri Krishna is perhaps the most celebrated hero in Hindu mythology and seems to be an historical figure. To uphold dharma he orchestrated the Mahabharata war. His teachings to his friend and disciple Arjuna during that war are immortalized in the *Bhagavad Gita*.

Kriya – action; cleansing practice (shatkarma); practice of kriya yoga.

Krodha – anger, aggression.

Kumbhaka – internal or external retention of the breath.

Kundalini – the evolutionary energy in a human being; spiritual energy; Devi described as the potential energy of a human being dormant in mooladhara chakra, which, when awakened, awakens the chakras, resulting in progressive enlightenment.

Kundalini yoga – path of yoga which awakens the dormant spiritual force, kundalini. See Kundalini.

Laghava, laghavatvam – the fifth limb of Sage Gheranda's saptanga yoga; lightness of body.

Lakshya – direction, aim.

Lauliki – see Nauli.

Laya yoga – literally, union by absorption; yoga of conscious dissolution of individuality.

Lila – literally, 'play'; activity of prakriti and its three gunas.

Linga, lingam – symbol; a naturally formed oval stone; often means Shivalingam. See Shivalingam.

Lota – pot.

Mada – arrogance.

Maha prana – prana in its cosmic unmanifest aspect.

Mahabharata – epic of ancient India said to be composed by Sage Veda Vyasa, involving the history and consequences of the great battle between the Kaurava and Pandava princes. It consists of eighteen sections and the *Bhagavad Gita* is a part of it.

Mala – impurity; dirt; impurity of mind such as lust, greed, anger.

Manas – finite mind, rational mind; the mind concerned with senses, thought and counter-thought; perception, intelligence.

Manas shakti – mental energy; one of the four parts of the antahkarana or inner instrument.

Mandala – circular symbolic pictorial depiction of cosmic power and/or the human psyche.

Manipura chakra – literally, 'city of jewels'; psychic/pranic centre situated in the spine behind the navel; associated with the solar plexus and digestive organs and mentally with willpower; source of vitality and energy.

Manomaya kosha – mental sheath or body; mental sphere of life and awareness.

Mantra – words of power; sound vibrations which liberate the mind when repeated.

Matsarya – envy; jealousy.

Maya – means by which Brahman creates the phenomenal world; power of creation; illusive power; in Vedanta philosophy, the two powers of maya are: 1. the power of veiling, and 2. the power of projection; in Samkhya philosophy, another name for Prakriti; comprised of e.g. annamaya, comprised of food (anna).

Mayurasana – peacock pose; an advanced yogasana which exerts pressure on the abdominal region.

Moha – delusion; infatuation.

Moksha – liberation from the cycles of birth and death and the illusion of maya.

Moola – literally, 'base' or 'root'; anus and rectum.

Moola bandha – perineum contraction; contraction of the perineal body in the male and the cervix in the female body; technique used for locating and awakening mooladhara chakra.

Mooladhara chakra – the lowest psychic/pranic centre in the human body; situated in the perineal floor in men and the cervix in women; associated physically with the coccygeal plexus, excretory and reproductive organs, and mentally with the instinctive nature; spiritually it is the seat of kundalini.

Mudra – literally, 'gesture'; psychic, emotional, devotional, and aesthetic gestures; attitudes of energy intended to link individual pranic force with universal or cosmic force.

Mukti – release, liberation, final absolution of the consciousness from the chain of birth and death and from the illusion of maya.

Nada – sound; subtle sound or vibration created by the union of the Shiva and Shakti tattwas; the first manifestation of the unmanifest Absolute.

Nada yoga – the process of penetrating deeper and deeper into the nature of one's own reality by listening to subtle inner sounds.

Nadabrahmananda, Swami – disciple of Swami Sivananda and an accomplished nada yogi.

Nadi – flow; a river or channel of energy; psychic current; subtle channel in the pranic body, conducting the flow of shakti; comparable to the meridians of acupuncture.

Nadi shodhana pranayama – nadi purification; a pranayama designed to purify and balance the two main energy flows of the body, ida and pingala nadis.

Nadi shuddhi – cleansing of the pathways of prana, nadis.

Nasikagra drishti – nosetip gazing; a practice to stimulate mooladhara chakra.

Nauli – abdominal massaging; one of the shatkarmas in which the rectus abdominis muscles are contracted and isolated vertically.

Neti – one of the shatkarmas; nasal cleansing with saline water (jala neti), a waxed string (sutra neti) or other elements.

Niranjana – stainless.

Nirguna – without quality or attribute; formless.

Nirguna dhyana – meditation without form.

Nirlipta, nirliptam – the seventh limb of Sage Gheranda's saptanga yoga; the state of being unattached.

Nirmala – pure, sacred.

Om – See Aum

Padahastasana – hand to foot pose; a forward bending asana in the standing position.

Padmasana – lotus pose; classical meditative posture.
Pancha – five.
Pancha prana – five major divisions of the pranic energy located in the physical body.
Pancha tattwa – the five elements, consisting of ether or space (akasha), gases or air (vayu), light or fire (agni), liquids or water (apas) and solids or earth (prithvi).
Paschimottanasana – back stretching pose; a forward bending posture.
Patanjali, Sage – author of the *Yoga Sutras*; an ancient rishi who codified the system of raja yoga, including ashtanga yoga.
Pawanmuktasana – a group of asanas that remove any blockages preventing free flow of energy in the body and mind; three groups of asanas: the anti-rheumatic group, the digestive/abdominal group, and the energy block releasing group (shakti bandhas).
Pingala nadi – a major pranic channel in the body which conducts the dynamic pranic force manifesting as prana shakti from the right side of mooladhara chakra, criss-crossing the spine through the major chakras to the right side of ajna chakra; associated with the mundane realm of experience and externalized awareness; also called surya nadi as the solar energy flows through it.
Pitta – bile, one of the three humours (doshas) described in ayurveda.
Pooja – worship.
Poorna – whole, complete, full.
Poornima – the day of the full moon.
Prana – vital energy force sustaining life and creation, permeating the whole of creation and existing in both the macrocosmos and microcosmos.
Prana shakti – energy; dynamic solar force governing the dimension of matter; energy flow related to externalization of mind; the force of prana.
Prana vayu – pranic air current; also refers to a specific current, one of the pancha pranas or vayus, located in

the thoracic region, from the throat to the diaphragm, responsible for processes of inspiration and absorption.

Pranamaya kosha – energy sheath, or vital pranic body; the sheath covering the self which is composed of pranic vibration and the rhythm of pranic forces.

Pranayama – a series of techniques using the breath to control the flow of prana within the body.

Pranotthana – awakening of the pranas in the different nadis and chakras; a stage of awakening preparatory to kundalini awakening.

Pratyahara – restraining the sensory and motor organs; withdrawal and emancipation of the mind from the domination of the senses and sensual objects; training the senses to follow the mind within; fifth stage of ashtanga yoga described by Sage Patanjali in the *Yoga Sutras*.

Pratyaksha – the sixth limb of Sage Gheranda's saptanga yoga; inner perception; inner acceptance; present before the eyes, visible, perceptible, clear.

Pratyaya – seeds or impressions in the field of consciousness which do not disappear even in the first stages of samadhi; content of mind.

Puranas – eighteen ancient texts containing the earliest mythology of the tantric and vedic traditions.

Raja yoga – the supreme yoga; union through control of the mental processes and concentration of the mind; the most authoritative text is Sage Patanjali's *Yoga Sutras* which contains ashtanga yoga, the eightfold path.

Rajas – one of the three gunas or attributes; dynamism; state of activity; creativity combined with full ego involvement.

Ramana Maharshi – (1879–1950) a renowned jnana yogi and enlightened sage who taught mainly through silence; establisher of the path of self-enquiry.

Rechaka – the process of exhalation in pranayama; emptying of the lungs.

Rishi – seer; realized sage; one who contemplates or meditates on the Self.

Sadhaka – one who practises sadhana; a spiritual aspirant.

Sadhana – spiritual practice or discipline performed regularly.

Sadhu – good or holy person, sage, saint.

Saguna – with qualities (gunas).

Saguna dhyana – meditation with form.

Sahasrara chakra – 'thousand-petalled lotus'; abode of Shiva or superconsciousness; highest chakra or psychic centre, it symbolizes the threshold between the psychic and spiritual realms and is located at the crown of the head.

Samadhi – the culmination of meditation, state of oneness of the mind with the object of concentration and the universal consciousness; self-realization; the eighth stage of raja yoga.

Samana vayu – one of the five pancha pranas or vayus, it is located between the navel and the diaphragm; it flows from side to side and controls the digestion.

Samskara – mental impression stored in the subtle body as an archetype; the impressions which condition one's nature, causing one to react or respond in a certain way.

Saptanga yoga – the seven limbs of yoga described by Sage Gheranda in *Gheranda Samhita*, viz. purification, firmness, steadiness, patience, lightness, inner perception and non-involvement.

Sattwa – one of the three gunas, or attributes of nature; state of luminosity, harmony, equilibrium and purity.

Shabda – sound; perceptible sound; object of the sense of hearing and property of space; word.

Shabda Brahman – the form of Brahman as sound.

Shakti – primal energy; manifest consciousness; power, ability, capacity, strength, energy; counterpart of Shiva; the moving power of nature and consciousness; in Hindu mythology Shakti is often symbolized as a divine woman.

Shakti nadi – an energy flow which starts from the right side of the anus and goes up to mooladhara and swadhisthana chakras where it joins pingala nadi. See Nadi.

Shambhavi mudra – eyebrow centre gazing; psychic attitude focused on Shiva (Supreme Consciousness).

Shankha – conch.

Shatkarma – the six hatha yoga techniques of purification: neti, dhauti, basti, nauli, kapalbhati and trataka.

Shavasana – the corpse pose; a relaxation posture.

Sheetali pranayama – cooling breath; a cooling pranayama.

Sheetkari pranayama – hissing breath; a cooling pranayama.

Shiva – state of pure consciousness, individual and cosmic, original source of yoga; Lord of yogis; auspicious, benevolent one; name of the god of the Hindu trinity who is entrusted with the work of destruction; destroyer of the ego and duality.

Shivalingam – black oval-shaped stone; symbol of Lord Shiva; symbol of consciousness.

Shivaratri – 14th night of the dark lunar fortnight in the month of Phalguna (which falls in February or March).

Shodhana, shodhanam – first limb of Sage Gheranda's saptanga yoga; purification.

Shoonya – void, state of transcendental consciousness; space behind the eyebrow centre.

Siddha – an adept or perfected person; one who has developed his/her psychic and pranic capacity to the point of mastery.

Siddha yoni asana – classical meditation posture, the male equivalent is siddhasana.

Siddhasana – accomplished pose; classical cross-legged meditation posture.

Siddhi – perfection; enhanced pranic and psychic capacity; paranormal or supernormal accomplishment; control of mind and prana; eight supernatural powers obtained by yogis as a result of long practice.

Sphatika – crystal.

Sri Yantra – geometric diagram representing the divine 'female' energy, or shakti.

Sthairya, sthairyam – the third limb of Sage Gheranda's saptanga yoga; steadiness.

Sthoola sharira – gross, physical body; annamaya kosha.

Sukhasana – easy pose; a cross-legged meditation asana.

Sukshma sharira – subtle body composed of pranamaya, manomaya and vijnanamaya koshas; part of the subconscious which manifests in the dream state.

Surya namaskara – salutations to the sun; a dynamic series of twelve postures.

Surya shakti – solar force; vital pranic energy; pingala nadi.

Sushumna – central energy flow (nadi) in the spine; it conducts the kundalini or spiritual force from mooladhara chakra to sahasrara chakra; the main energy flow related to transcendental awareness; situated in the spinal cord of the human body, it opens when balance is achieved between ida and pingala nadis.

Sutra – thread; condensed statements strung together to give an outline of a philosophy, such as the *Yoga Sutras* of Sage Patanjali.

Swadhisthana chakra – literally, 'one's own abode'; second psychic/pranic centre; located in the coccyx; associated with the sacral plexus and governing the urogenital system; the storehouse of subconscious impressions.

Swara – breathing cycle; flow of the breath in the nostrils.

Swara yoga – science of the breathing cycle; the system of yoga using understanding and management of the breathing cycle as a means to attain self-realization.

Swatmarama, Yogi – literally, 'one who revels within oneself'; the author of *Hatha Yoga Pradipika*, a classical text book in hatha yoga.

Swayambhu – self-existing.

Tadasana – palm tree pose; a standing asana in which the body is stretched upward; used in shankhaprakshalana.

Tamas – one of the three gunas or attributes of nature; inertia, stability; ignorance, darkness; unwillingness to change.

Tantra – most ancient universal science and culture which deals with the transition of human nature from the present level of evolution and understanding to a transcendental level of knowledge, experience and awareness; a particular path of sadhana including mantra, yantra and other esoteric practices.

Tattwa – 'that-ness'; true essential nature; an element, a primary substance; the five elements (space, air, fire, water and earth); another name for mahabhoota.

Tha – seed mantra of chandra shakti.

Tiryak bhujangasana – twisting cobra pose; a backward bending asana incorporating a spinal twist; used in shankhaprakshalana.

Tiryak tadasana – swaying palm tree pose; a side bending asana; used in shankhaprakshalana.

Trataka – one of the shatkarmas; a technique of gazing steadfastly upon an object such as a candle flame, black dot or yantra with unblinking eyes.

Tridosha – refers to all of the three doshas or humours in the body. See Dosha.

Trikonasana – triangle pose; a side-bending standing asana from the stretching category.

Udana vayu – one of the five pancha pranas or vayus, it is located in the extremities of the body: arms, legs and head; it flows with a spiraling motion and rises up the throat entering the head; it controls the sensory and motor organs.

Udarakarshanasana – abdominal stretch pose; one of the shakti bandha asanas; used in shankhaprakshalana.

Uddhava Gita – classical text giving teachings of Sri Krishna to his friend and disciple, Uddhava.

Uddiyana bandha – abdominal retraction lock; drawing in of the abdomen towards the backbone after exhaling.

Ujjayi pranayama – a subtle pranayama often used during meditation; the psychic breath.

Upanishads – the philosophical portion of the Vedas, traditionally one hundred and eight in number, containing intimate dialogues and discussions between guru and disciple on the nature of the Absolute and the path leading towards it; literally, 'to sit near and listen' (to the spiritual teacher); regarded as the source of Vedanta, Yoga and Samkhya philosophies.

Upasana – personalized form of worship.

Utkatasana – unyielding pose; a squatting pose.

Utthanpadasana – stretched leg pose; a forward bending asana in sitting position.

Vajra nadi – the nadi starting on the left side of the anus governing the sexual organs and processes, the digestive system, and related to the sciatic nerve.

Vajrasana – thunderbolt pose; a kneeling meditative posture.

Vajroli mudra – contraction and release of the male urinary passage to stimulate swadhisthana chakra and promote brahmacharya; controlling the emissions during sexual intercourse according to hatha yoga texts.

Vasana – subtle impressions which are the seeds of desires.

Vastra – cloth.

Vata – wind, gas; one of the three humours (doshas) described in ayurveda. See Dosha.

Vedas – ancient texts revealed to the sages and saints of India, explaining and regulating every aspect of life from the Supreme Reality to worldly affairs; four in number: Rig, Yajur, Sama, Atharva, which are further divided into the Samhita, Brahmana, Aranyaka and Upanishads; the oldest books in the library of mankind, parts of them revealed to sages and seers before 5,000 BC.

Vijnanamaya kosha – astral or psychic (higher mental) sheath or body; one of the sheaths of the soul, consisting of the principle of intellect or buddhi, the subtler level of our own existence with its vision, intuition, wisdom and power of understanding; the covering of the self which is made of knowledge.

Vikara – toxin; modification or change, generally with reference to the modifications of mind; impurities (in Samkhya philosophy) which are evolved from a previous source or from prakriti.

Vikshepa – dissipation; the tossing of mind which obstructs concentration.

Vishnu – vedic deity; the second deity of the Hindu trinity (Brahma, Vishnu, Shiva), entrusted with the preservation of the universe, a duty which obliges him to appear in several incarnations; Supreme Consciousness.

Vishuddhi chakra – literally, 'centre of purification', the psychic/pranic centre located at the level of the throat pit or the thyroid gland; it is the psychic centre particularly connected with purification and communication.

Vritti – a modification arising in the mind related to a thought pattern; a particular state or condition.

Vyana vayu – one of the pancha pranas or vayus; the reserve of pranic energy pervading the entire body.

Yantra – a geometric symbol of cosmic power designed to unleash the hidden potential energy and consciousness; used in meditation and concentration practices.

Yoga – union; the root is yuj, meaning 'to join', ' to yoke'; a system of practice leading to a state of union between the individual and universal awareness; practices, philosophy and lifestyle to achieve peace, power and spiritual wisdom as well as perfect health, a sound mind and a balanced personality; one of the six main systems of Indian philosophy.

Yoga nidra – psychic sleep; practice in which the body sleeps while the mind remains aware as its movements are guided and quietened by instructions, inducing deep relaxation of body, mind and emotions.

Yoga Sutras – ancient authoritative text on raja yoga by Sage Patanjali.

Yoga Upanishads – a group of approximately twenty-two Upanishads more specifically concerned with yoga.

Yogi – an adept of yoga; follower of the yoga system of philosophy and practice.

Yoni mudra – attitude of the womb or source; a hand mudra; also another name for shanmuki mudra.

General Index